Preventing and Managing

Back Pain

During Pregnancy

Preventing and Managing

Back Pain

During Pregnancy

by

Alicia M. Silva, MSPT

The instructions and advice presented in this book are in no way meant as a substitute for medical care. It is therefore essential to discuss any back pain you are experiencing with your physician, obstetrician, or midwife prior to following any recommendations in this book. You should get clearance from your health care provider before commencing this, or any exercise program. If you are having a high-risk pregnancy including any complications resulting in bed rest or restricted activity, do not perform any exercise without the consent of your physician/midwife.

Doing exercises incorrectly can result in injury, and any exercises that cause pain should be avoided.

Some forms of back pain may not respond well to exercise and may require professional treatment by a physical therapist or other specialist. In some cases, severe back pain may be due to a more serious problem, contractions, or possibly labor. Consult with your physician or midwife regarding your symptoms and appropriate treatment options.

Library of Congress Cataloging-in Publication Data
2004094673

ISBN 0-9755826-2-3

Printed in the United States of America

To Matt, Andrew, and Abrielle
. . . for everyday.

Acknowledgements

There are so many people who helped me along the way as this book evolved. I would like to recognize all of my patients who always keep me thinking and generating new ideas. The concept for this book came from working with pregnant and post-partum women with back pain who did not have a comprehensive resource available to reference.

I greatly appreciate the time and expertise of Lorraine Hamwey, Layout Designer, for all of her help and support throughout this project. I would also like to thank John Hamwey, Graphic Designer, for his consultation and contributions toward image editing, and for his patience and expertise in assisting with the book cover design. Thanks also go to my Editorial Consultants, Jonathan Gerson, MBA and Elizabeth Remke, MSPT for their feedback and input. Special thanks also go to Dr. Jennifer Daman, Jennifer McSweeney, CNM and Dr. Marcie Richardson for taking the time to give their critique and suggestions.

I would never have completed this book without the love, support, and wisdom of my husband, Dr. Matt. His efforts to inspire, critique, edit, design, and proofread (again and again and again) made all the difference.

CONTENTS

FOREWORD

Up to 80% of women will experience back pain at some point during pregnancy, most commonly in the third trimester, due to weight gain and postural changes. Many women accept pain as just one of the many "side effects" of pregnancy, along with morning sickness and swollen ankles; however, back pain should not be considered a normal part of pregnancy. This book is designed to teach you how to prevent and manage back pain. As a physical therapist, I have treated many women both during and after their pregnancies. Not until my own pregnancies did I really appreciate what the pregnant body endures as it changes and prepares for childbirth. I have mild scoliosis (an abnormal curvature of the spine), with a history of upper and lower back problems, and I was extremely concerned about back pain during my pregnancies. However, by performing the appropriate exercises, moving my body safely, and listening to my body, I experienced happy, healthy, and "back-pain-free" pregnancies.

My pregnant patients, friends, and family, who have struggled with back pain, inspired me to write an easy to follow guide for its prevention and management. I hope you find this book a helpful tool both during and after your pregnancy.

I wish you superb health, happiness, and success throughout your pregnancy, labor, delivery, post-partum recovery, and motherhood.

Alicia Silva

Alicia Silva, MSPT

HOW TO USE THIS BOOK

If you have this book because you are experiencing pregnancy-related back pain, you are likely eager to take measures to be rid of your pain. I strongly encourage you to read the first five chapters, discussing the anatomy of the spine and causes of back pain during pregnancy, as it will provide you with a clearer understanding of how to manage back pain. Chapters 6–10 are the foundation for the Recommended Programs and provide detailed information on safe exercise during pregnancy, as well as specific exercises that are presented for back pain management. Having a thorough understanding of the safety guidelines and proper form will help to maximize the effectiveness of your efforts and help to ensure that you do not injure yourself.

Should you feel the urgency to skip ahead, you may refer directly to Chapter 12, Recommended Daily Programs, and select the program that pertains to your situation. There are specific programs for each trimester as well as programs based on the common problem areas during pregnancy. You will need to reference back to Chapters 7-10 to understand how to perform various exercises, but you will be able to get started more quickly. If you choose this approach, it will be very beneficial to go back and read the introductory materials to increase your likelihood of success with the program.

There are many strengthening, stretching, and postural exercises recommended throughout this book. It is not reasonable or necessary to complete all of the exercises every day. You can mix and match the various exercises in order to vary which muscle groups you work and help to prevent boredom. You might find one particular group of exercises makes you feel best and decide to maintain only those exercises. I encourage you to do whatever combination of exercises works best for you. As mentioned above, I have included several sample programs to give you ideas and help get you moving in the right direction.

The instructions and advice presented in this book are in no way meant as a substitute for medical care. It is therefore essential to discuss any back pain you are experiencing with your physician, obstetrician, or midwife prior to following any recommendations in this book. You should get clearance from your health care provider before commencing this, or any exercise program. If you are having a high-risk pregnancy including any complications resulting in bed rest or restricted activity, do not perform any exercise without the consent of your physician/midwife.

Doing exercises incorrectly can result in injury, and any exercises that cause pain should be avoided.

Some forms of back pain may not respond well to exercise and may require professional treatment by a physical therapist or other specialist. In some cases, severe back pain may be due to a more serious problem, contractions, or possibly labor. Consult with your physician or midwife regarding your symptoms and appropriate treatment options.

~1~

Introduction

The pregnant body is truly miraculous, adapting to accommodate a growing child and undergoing constant changes. Although pregnancy is generally a wonderful experience, there are several associated discomforts including: morning sickness, indigestion, varicose veins, leg cramps, fatigue, swelling, and hemorrhoids. Further, as many as 80% of women will experience back pain at some point during their pregnancies. The severity of this pain ranges from mild discomfort after standing for long periods, to debilitating pain that limits a woman's ability to function. This book is designed to decrease back pain by:

- Describing the basic anatomy of the spine
- Explaining the changes in the pregnant body that contribute to back pain
- Providing exercises that create a balance between the flexibility and stability of the muscles throughout the body to decrease back pain
- Educating women on how to move in safe ways to prevent and minimize strain to the spine

- Improving posture during pregnancy to reduce discomfort
- Preparing the body for the work of labor and delivery
- Aiding in post-partum recovery

The spine is an amazing structure that creates the framework for the entire body. It allows the body to move freely and with control, enabling us to perform everyday activities, hobbies, and sports. The various parts of the spine work together to provide the body with a high level of physical functioning. A brief description of the anatomy of the spine is included so you can visualize how and where problems might occur.

As you will learn from this book, the pregnant body loses joint stability due to hormonal changes that take place to allow the pelvis to spread as your baby grows. In addition, weight gain and the changing shape of the female body contribute to postural changes that can increase stress on the spine.

The key to minimizing pain within the unstable pregnant spine is to achieve optimal balance between muscle strength and flexibility. It is essential to strengthen key muscles around the spine (back, abdominal, pelvic floor, hip muscles) to provide some added stability and protection. It is also important to maintain good flexibility to prevent tight muscles from exerting excess force on less stable joints, which could result in discomfort. Improved flexibility also allows you to assume certain birthing positions, such as squatting, which can facilitate delivery.

Strength   Flexibility

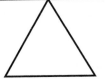

*Balance between strength and flexibility
is the key to a pain-free spine.*

Pregnant or not, a major factor that contributes to back pain is the imbalance in muscle strength and flexibility, coupled with poor postural habits. Muscles need to be strong to support the joints. Muscles must also be flexible so skeletal movements can occur without restrictions. As an introductory example, the abdominal muscles are a main stabilizer for the lower back. If the abdominals are weak, the lower back is vulnerable to injury because it is not well supported for strenuous activities. In addition, if lower back and hamstring muscles (back of the thigh) are inflexible, they will limit how far you can bend forward, and create more stress on the lower back. The majority of people I treat for back pain are living with this combination of muscle weakness in the abdominals and inflexibility in the hamstrings and lower back.

Poor posture, including slouching, repetitive bending, and incorrect lifting techniques, is another common cause of painful conditions of the spine. Pregnant women experience significant changes in their posture due to the increased weight distribution at the abdomen. If coupled with poor postural habits, they are at an even greater risk of injury. There are correct and incorrect ways to perform activities as basic as getting out of bed and lifting a two year old child. Learning how to perform these everyday tasks "correctly" will minimize strain to the back and improve the overall health of the spine.

It is important to remember that your body and your baby are changing and preparing over forty long weeks for the anxiously awaited birth. You must take time to prepare both mentally and physically for the challenge of pregnancy and childbirth. Beyond setting up the nursery and packing your hospital bags, as a mother-to-be you should also optimize your health in preparation for labor and delivery and the new responsibility of caring for a newborn. The exercises and techniques recommended in this book are beneficial not only for back pain prevention and management, but also to facilitate your labor and delivery. One study showed the following benefits of exercise during pregnancy[1]:

- Less need for cesarean surgery
- Lower pain medicine requirements
- Shorter duration of active labor
- 75% decreased need for operative intervention
- 50% less need to induce or stimulate labor
- 55% decreased episiotomy rate

Performing the recommended exercises can help you prevent and manage back pain and achieve a balance between stability and flexibility, which will help during pregnancy, labor, and delivery. It will also facilitate an easier post-partum recovery. With a new little one to nurture, the better you feel physically, the easier it will be to enjoy the time you spend caring for and getting to know your baby.

---

[1]Clapp JF 3rd. The course of labor after endurance exercise during pregnancy. Am J Obstet Gynecol. 1990 Dec;163(6 Pt 1):1799-805.

~2~

Anatomy
of the Spine

The spine is the center, or core, of the human body. It connects the extremities to the trunk, and provides stability to allow for smooth, coordinated movement. Although it is not necessary to have a thorough understanding of the anatomy of the spine, it is helpful to be familiar with its regions, natural curves, and functions.

CERVICAL SPINE

The cervical spine, or neck region, is comprised of seven bones (vertebrae) that start beneath the skull. These vertebrae connect the head to the shoulders and trunk, and support the head, which can weigh 9 to 11 pounds. The neck also allows for significant mobility, enabling you to look around at the world. The cervical spine naturally curves inward. The medical term for this is lordosis.

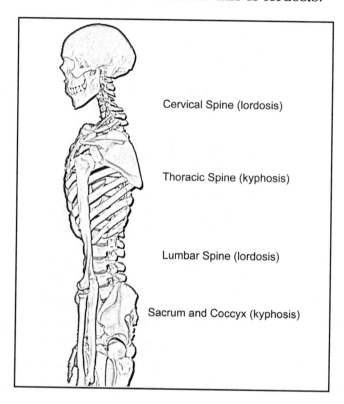

Cervical Spine (lordosis)

Thoracic Spine (kyphosis)

Lumbar Spine (lordosis)

Sacrum and Coccyx (kyphosis)

THORACIC SPINE

This region of the spine, known as the thorax, is made up of 12 vertebrae. Each vertebra is connected to a rib, which connects from the back of the spine to the front of the chest along the sternum, or breastbone. The eleventh and twelfth ribs do not attach to the sternum and are known as free ribs. This area of the spine has a role in breathing, as it must expand each time you inhale. The thoracic spine naturally curves outward. The medical term for this is kyphosis.

LUMBAR SPINE

The lumbar spine is made up of five large vertebrae. This region of the spine supports a large amount of the body's weight, allows mobility, and helps protect the abdominal organs. The lumbar spine naturally curves inward. Injury to the lumbar spine is prevalent during pregnancy due to postural changes that occur, resulting in an increased lordosis and excess strain on the lower back.

SACRUM AND COCCYX

The sacrum and coccyx form the base of the spine. The sacrum, consisting of five fused bones, is triangular in shape. It connects the spine to the pelvis, and forms the pelvic cavity, which houses the abdominal and pelvic organs and your growing baby. Beneath the sacrum is the coccyx, more commonly known as the tailbone. The sacrum and coccyx curve outward when viewed from the side.

THE PELVIC BONES AND
THE SACROILIAC (SI) JOINT

The pelvis is made up of two symmetrical bones, one on each side of the body. Each of these bones is comprised of an ilium, ischium, and pubic segment. The ilia are the bones you feel when you rest your hands on your waist. They form the top crest of the pelvis. The ischia are the "sit bones" under the buttock muscles and are the weight bearing bones when you are seated. The pubic bones are located in the front of the pelvis several inches below the navel.

Due to the complexity of the pelvis, it is simplist to list its many joints:

- The true hip joint: connects the pelvis to the leg bone
- The sacroiliac joint: the point on each side of the pelvis where the sacrum meets the ilium
- The pubic symphysis: the joint at the front of the pelvis where the two pubic bones meet

The junction of the pelvic bones with the sacrum and coccyx creates the pelvic cavity which houses the bladder, bowel, uterus and most significantly, your growing baby.

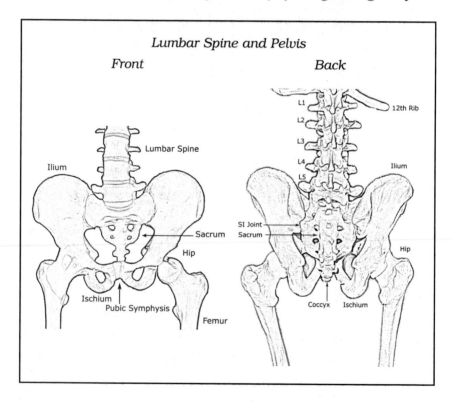

Lumbar Spine and Pelvis

NEUTRAL SPINE POSTURE

As mentioned above, each region of the spine has a natural curve inward (lordosis) or outward (kyphosis). When all of these natural curves are present, the spine is considered to be in "neutral" position. The spine is strongest and least vulnerable to injury when in its neutral position. Therefore, when lifting, reaching, doing housework, or even getting in and out of bed, the spine should be kept in its neutral alignment to prevent injury.

When the spinal curves become excessive or diminished, the spine is no longer in neutral alignment. The spine attempts to compensate for changes in posture to maintain an upright view of the world. If for example, your lower back arches excessively, your head would be looking up to the ceiling. No person would choose to go about their day looking up. It would make driving, working, and eating almost impossible. In order to compensate for this, the upper back might round forward excessively bringing the head forward, allowing you to still view the world on the horizon. When the lower back arches excessively, the abdominals get over-stretched. When the upper

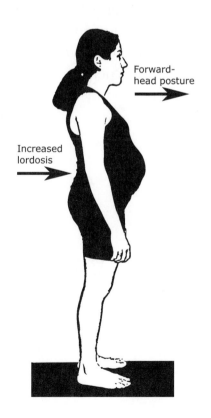

Forward-head posture →

Increased lordosis →

back is excessively rounded, the muscles and ligaments in the upper back get overstretched. These structures, when overstretched, weaken and can easily be injured. In this instance, the lower back, upper back, and neck are susceptible to injury; and the longer this poor posture occurs, the greater the chance that a painful condition will develop.

It is therefore important to maintain "neutral spine" posture when going about your day-to-day activities in order to prevent weakness and injury. If you were to look around at people on the street, chances are the majority would not be moving with neutral spine posture. Slouching is easy, because the muscles don't have to work; instead, the body relies on ligaments rather than muscles for support. It is crucial to try to maintain good posture in order to prevent spinal dysfunction. It is even more important during pregnancy, due to all the changes in the body as your baby grows. We will cover body mechanics to elucidate specific exercises and positions for healthy, neutral spine posture in Chapter 10.

~3~

Putting the Pieces Together

How the Regions Are Connected

The spine is a complex structure comprised of the vertebrae, spinal cord, nerves, discs, bones, ligaments, and muscles. Each component plays a crucial role in human movement and posture and must function properly for a healthy spine. Putting the pieces together will provide a comprehensive picture of the spine.

Spinal Cord and Nerves

There is a circular opening (foramen) in each vertebra through which runs the spinal cord, the bundle of nerves that sends messages to and from the brain. The bony ring created by the vertebrae protects the spinal cord. The nerves that travel to the extremities branch off from the spinal cord between the vertebral joints. The spinal cord and nerves send messages from the brain to the body, such as "put my hand on my belly so I can feel the baby kicking." They also send messages from the body back to the brain to be processed. For example, if you've been standing in line at your favorite store too long, your body might send a signal of pain to the brain, which would prompt you to move and change your position.

Discs

The vertebrae are separated by discs, which act as shock absorbers for the spine. The discs cushion the bones and help absorb stress, especially from high impact activities. With spinal movement, the discs move as well. When a person bends forward, pressure is put on the front of the disc, which can result in the disc being displaced out the back. When a person arches backwards, the disc moves forward. A simple analogy is to think of the disc as a jelly donut. When you press one end of the donut, jelly will squirt out the other end. The same can be visualized for the disc. When the disc gets displaced and doesn't return to its ideal position, it is considered a bulging disc. A bulging disc, which most commonly bulges out the back of the spine, is generally the result of years of bad posture and muscle imbalances. The one time you bend forward and rupture a disc, is usually the last straw in a process of gradual wear, tear, and trauma. Although a common source of back pain in the general population, disc problems are rare during pregnancy.

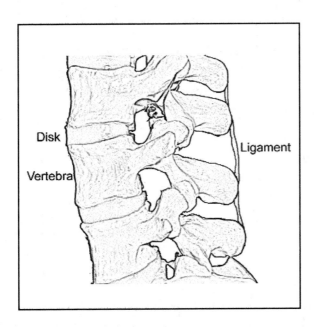

LIGAMENTS

Throughout the body, every bone is connected to adjacent bones by ligaments, bands of connective tissue that give stability to the joints. In the spine, ligaments connect the vertebrae to each other, and to the ribs, the pelvis, and the skull. Ligaments are designed to limit excessive joint motion. Ligaments can be thought of like rubber bands. They stretch elastically to accommodate movement. Towards the end of the normal range of motion, however, they become increasingly taut to prevent over-stretching. When over-stretched, a ligament goes beyond the point of elasticity and becomes deformed. It is unable to return to its original size, spraining the ligament. Due to hormonal changes that take place as your body prepares for the growth and birth of your baby, the ligaments become more lax and thus vulnerable to injury.

MUSCLES

There are muscles that travel along the front, back, and sides of the spine. A good balance between the strength and flexibility in these muscles is a key element in back pain prevention and management. Muscles give the body strength and allow bending, twisting, and arching motions to occur. When strong, they provide added stability to the joints.

The key stabilizers of the spine are the back, abdominal, and pelvic floor muscles. The back muscles act to extend the spine, as well as allow for rotation and side bending. Good back strength helps support and protect the many spinal joints, as well as maintain good posture.

The abdominals allow the spine to bend forward, rotate, and bend side to side. The abdominals, more so than the back muscles, must be strong to support and protect the spine, particularly the lumbopelvic regions. It is interesting to note that as your belly grows, the abdominal muscles get stretched very taut, naturally weakening them. Considering the abdominals play a major role in stabilizing the spine, this creates an obvious disadvantage for the spine, especially in light of ligamentous and postural changes.

The pelvic floor muscles are located in the saddle area (if you were to sit on a saddle, the area that contacts it is referred to as the pelvic floor region) and connect the pubic bone in the front to the coccyx in the back. The pelvic floor supports the pelvic organs, including the bladder, which is why weakness in these muscles can cause incontinence, or leakage of urine when you cough or sneeze. In addition, the pelvic floor supports the weight of your growing baby.

The large leg muscles of the buttocks, hips, and thighs also help stabilize the pelvis. It is therefore important to have good strength in these muscle groups to support the pelvis as you go about your everyday life, especially during pregnancy when your body is changing at such a rapid pace.

Good flexibility in the muscle groups discussed above is equally important for a pain free spine. When the muscles are flexible, they allow the body to move without restrictions or unnecessary limitations. However, when these muscles are tight, they can pull the bones into sub-optimal alignment, placing undue stress on the joints. This can result in pain as well as poor posture.

CHAPTER CONCLUSION

With all of these structures in the spine, it may seem apparent how vulnerable it is to injury. Like many household appliances, the more parts something has, the more likely one component will break. Unfortunately, there is not an owner's manual for or a warrantee on the human spine, so care must be taken to protect it and perform appropriate maintenance on it.

The next chapter will explain why the back is particularly vulnerable during pregnancy, followed by a discussion of the maintenance recommendations needed for a pain free pregnancy.

~4~

Understanding Back Pain During Pregnancy

Back pain during pregnancy can arise in any of the regions of the spine previously discussed and can vary from minor discomfort to debilitating pain. Lumbar spine and sacroiliac joint pain are the most common problem areas, due to changes in joint stability, body weight and shape, and posture. Although the changes that occur in the pregnant woman are fascinating to watch and feel, they can wreak havoc on the body — especially the spine.

JOINT LAXITY

Ligaments connect and stabilize the joints throughout the body. As mentioned previously, ligaments have an elastic

Factors Contributing to Pregnancy-Related Back Pain

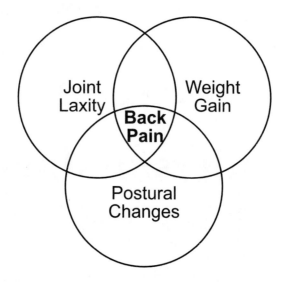

property and are designed to prevent excess joint motion. During pregnancy, the ligaments loosen due to a hormone called Relaxin, which literally relaxes the ligaments throughout the body. The increase in the ligaments' laxity results in decreased joint stability, and is necessary for pregnancy and childbirth.

The baby sits within the pelvic cavity, which in its normal (non-pregnant) state is not large enough to house the growing uterus and baby. As the baby grows, the pelvic cavity must expand to allow space for the baby, placenta, and amniotic fluid. The pelvic joints are generally considered to be very stable; however, in response to the growing child and in preparation for delivery, the ligaments that stabilize these joints must be looser. Relaxin allows the ligaments around the sacroiliac joints and pubic symphysis to relax, which permits the joints to open. Although this is a necessary change, the laxity and excess mobility in the pelvis can increase the risk of spraining one of these joints. If you have ever turned or rolled your ankle, you already understand the pain associated with an injury to a ligament. The result is swelling, pain, weakness, and loss of function. During pregnancy, an activity such as twisting at the waist to reach for something can be enough to cause a sprain to the vulnerable ligaments of the lower back. This is why it is recommended to avoid activities that involve rotation of the spine, such as tennis or golf.

Further, it should be noted that the effect of Relaxin is systemic; that is, it does not isolate itself to the pelvic joints. It affects all the joints from head to toe. It is important to keep this in mind, as it is easier to sprain a joint, such as your ankle or knee, with lesser impact or force than you might expect. Ligamentous changes alone are not the cause of back pain during pregnancy; in conjunction with weight gain and postural changes, the spine is quite vulnerable as will be described in the following sections.

WEIGHT GAIN

The most obvious change in the pregnant woman's body is her changing shape as her baby grows. It is a spectacular sight to see the unmistakable protruding abdomen, and to watch a woman rub it as she feels her baby squirming, kicking, or hiccupping inside. The growing belly is what gets her noticed, and it is amazing the way others respond to it. Loved ones, acquaintances, even strangers, feel compelled to pat or rub it, often without asking permission. Pregnancy appears to be the one instance in this culture, where a protruding abdomen is considered beautiful and admirable. And it truly is.

There are guidelines for healthy weight gain during pregnancy. Gaining too little weight jeopardizes the health of the baby, who may not receive adequate nourishment. Excess weight gain can predispose a woman to complications such as gestational diabetes and back pain as well as decrease the odds of her returning to her pre-pregnancy weight. The American College of Obstetricians and Gynecologists recommends that pregnant women gain between 25 and 35 pounds. For women who are overweight, 15-25 pounds is recommended. For underweight women, the goal for weight gain is 28 to 40 pounds. For women carrying twins, 35-45 pounds is considered healthy. If you are eating a well balanced diet and exercising and you gain beyond the recommended weight, do not panic or become obsessed. Discuss your concerns with your health care provider to rule out any problems, and continue with your healthy lifestyle. I was surprised during my first pregnancy when my 5 foot 2 inch frame gained 42 pounds despite eating right and exercising. I had no back pain or other complications, and returned to my pre-pregnancy weight within two months.

The rapid weight gain and work of carrying an extra 25+ pounds over a period of 6-9 months (weight gain in the first trimester is generally minimal) is stressful to the body, which is used to a significantly lower weight. It results in greater load and impact on the joints, which are already more lax, increasing the risk of sprains or strains. Consider also that one study has shown that non-pregnant women who have a larger waist size have higher incidences of lower back pain.[1] The pregnant woman certainly has a larger waist, which may increase her risk of low back pain.

It makes sense that most women experience back pain in the third trimester, due to increased weight gain and the position of the baby. These factors, coupled with lax ligaments, predispose the pregnant woman to postural changes that cause dysfunction in the spine. Avoiding excess weight gain can help minimize additional stress to the joints and the extent of postural dysfunction she will experience. However, keep in mind that pregnancy is not a time to diet, as the body requires an additional 300 calories per day. Adequate caloric intake is a priority for a healthy pregnancy and baby. Making healthy food choices and keeping active should be all you need to do to gain the appropriate weight.

POSTURAL CHANGES

It is important to define and understand the body's center of gravity in order to appreciate how the changing shape of the pregnant body will affect posture. The center of gravity of an object is the point around which all of the object's weight is evenly distributed. The simplest example is a circle, whose center of gravity is in the middle. In the non-pregnant person standing upright, the body's center of gravity is roughly located at the position of the navel halfway between the front and back (i.e., in the middle of your midsection). In young children, whose heads are still disproportionately

---

[1]Han TS, Schouten JS, Lean ME, Seidell JC. The prevalence of low back pain and associations with body fatness, fat distribution and height. Int J Obes Relat Metab Disord. 1997 Jul;21(7):600-7.

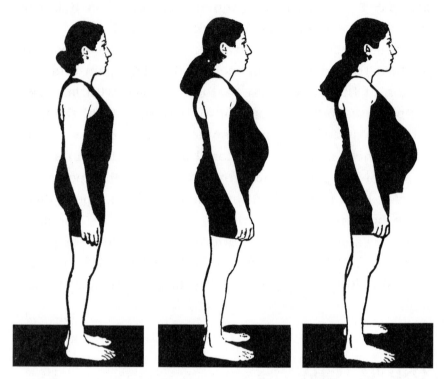

Posture at 12 weeks, 24 weeks, and 36 weeks of Pregnancy

Note increased arch in lower back and forward head and shoulders as pregnancy progresses.

larger, the center of gravity is higher up towards the chest because of the extra weight of the head. This higher center of gravity is what makes a toddler's balance unsteady.

Imagine you are carrying a very large watermelon at waist level. The weight of the watermelon pulls you forward. To maintain your balance, you would tend to lean backwards, arching the lower back, to keep your center of gravity in a location that prevents you from falling over. Similarly, in the pregnant woman, the majority of the weight gained is situated in the front of the belly. This shifts the woman's center of gravity forward, which would tend to make her lean forward. To compensate for this so that she still stands up straight, the pregnant woman tends to over arch her lower back, and excessively round her upper back and head forward. This change in posture puts the spine out of neutral alignment and into a position that is at risk of injury.

STRESS

Stress in not included as one of the major causative factors for back pain during pregnancy, although most health professionals agree that they are related. In response to stress the body releases hormones, which increase your heart rate and blood pressure, speed your rate of breathing, and activate muscle fibers. Pregnancy can sometimes be a stressful time as the body changes and decisions regarding parenting, finances, career, and child care loom. Do your best to identify your stressors and attempt to minimize them. Try to slow down, pamper yourself, or find a relaxing activity, such as yoga or meditation. Leading a balanced, healthy lifestyle, including proper nutrition, exercise, and rest, can effectively minimize stress.

CHAPTER CONCLUSION

In summary, joint instability, weight gain, and postural changes alone do not necessarily predispose an individual to back pain. This trio of factors has a cumulative effect on the pregnant woman and makes her more likely to experience back pain. Women are most likely to encounter problems during the third trimester, when weight gain is greatest, resulting in more strain on lax joints, and increased postural changes. Although these processes all occur during pregnancy as the body prepares for the arrival of the baby, the woman is not without options. She can maintain a good balance of strength and flexibility to minimize stress to the joints, exercise and eat right to prevent excess weight gain, and use good posture and safe body movements to minimize postural dysfunction. These combined techniques can help effectively prevent and manage back pain.

~5~

Locations of Back Pain During Pregnancy

Back pain is a nonspecific term that describes many different conditions of the spine. Back pain affects up to 85% of people at some point in their lives, and as explained previously, often impacts the pregnant woman due to the changes in her body. The common types of back pain during pregnancy will be discussed, as well as techniques for prevention and management.

SACROILIAC PAIN

The sacroiliac (SI) joints can be felt as the "dimples" in the left and right lower back. These joints connect the spine to the pelvis, and are a common source of back pain during pregnancy. The pain is typically unilateral (on one side), and can be very localized to the joint. However, it is possible to feel pain referred to the buttock or into the leg on the same side. The SI joint can be stressed by excessive or sudden bending, arching, or twisting of the spine. These motions can cause the pelvis or sacrum to move and get "stuck" out of neutral alignment. The pregnant woman also tends to stand duck-toed (toes pointing outward), which compresses the SI joints and can aggravate them. Another contributing factor to SI pain is muscle tightness in the leg muscles, specifically the hamstring, piriformis, and iliopsoas. Gentle stretching, strengthening, and postural exercises can help prevent and manage SI joint pain.

LOW BACK PAIN

Low back pain, in this case, refers to pain in the lumbar spine. Most commonly, the pregnant woman experiences pain at the lowest segments of the lumbar spine due to postural changes resulting in excessive extension in the lower back. The joints get compressed, resulting in pain and inflammation. The pain can be localized to the center of the lower back or may travel to the sides of the waist due to associated muscle spasm. Pain can also radiate to the buttocks or lower extremities, due to irritation of the nerves in this region. This low back pain can be managed by stretching, strengthening, posture correction, avoiding excess weight gain, and moving the body in a safe way.

SCIATICA

Sciatica is a condition resulting from irritation of the sciatic nerve. This nerve travels from the lower back, through the piriformis muscle in the buttock, and down the back of the leg to the foot. Sciatica is often felt as pain or burning in the buttock and/or the back of the leg. There can be numbness and tingling associated with sciatica. Bending, sitting slouched, and sitting with legs extended straight usually aggravate this condition. Sciatic pain is typically on one side.

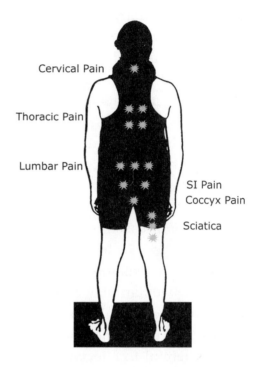

The sciatic nerve can be irritated by a disc rubbing against it, but disc bulging is very rare during pregnancy. (Typically disc bulging results from excess bending and poor posture, but it should also be noted that excess weight, vibration from driving, and smoking also exacerbate a disc condition.) The sciatic nerve can also be irritated if the buttock muscles, specifically the piriformis, are tight. Since the sciatic nerve travels between the fibers of the piriformis, if the muscle lacks flexibility it can put pressure on the sciatic nerve, causing symptoms. As mentioned previously, however, the low back and the SI joint can also refer pain to the buttock and back of the leg. In the absence of weakness or loss of bladder or bowel function, the management of all of these conditions is with similar exercises, as well as proper posture and body mechanics.

PUBIC SYMPHYSIS

The pubic symphysis is the joint at the front of the pelvis. It is a relatively immobile joint, but due to Relaxin, this joint becomes more mobile during pregnancy. Although uncommon, separation of the pubic symphysis may occur during pregnancy. Typical symptoms include pain in the region above the pubic bones with radiating pain to the back of the legs. There may be associated SI joint pain as well, as the SI joints tend to get compressed when the pubic symphysis separates. Pain is often worse when walking, and in severe cases, the woman may require a walker in order to ambulate any great distances. A pregnancy support brace can be helpful in alleviating pain, but for some women a brace may cause more discomfort. It is important to avoid stretching the inner thighs (positions tht spread your legs apart) in the presence of this condition, as it can

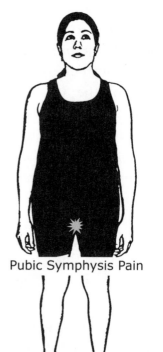

Pubic Symphysis Pain

exacerbate the pain and potentially worsen the separation.

The pubic symphysis spreads as the baby's head travels through the pelvic outlet, and sometimes it separates excessively during delivery. If this occurs, women can experience symptoms similar to those mentioned above. Physical therapy can be beneficial for treating this condition post-partum. If you think you are experiencing pubic symphysis pain, it is important to discuss your symptoms with your health care provider.

Coccyx

The coccyx, or tailbone, is another potential site of pain for the pregnant woman. Like the other vertebrae, the coccyx is connected to the spine via ligaments, which become lax. The coccyx becomes more mobile and can move out of its ideal alignment, in a hinge like motion, causing pain. The pain typically results from sitting in a slouched position, which places excess pressure on the tailbone.

Awareness of your sitting posture is one key factor in preventing coccygeal pain. When seated, make sure to scoot back in the chair and sit upright (this prevents slouching and coccyx sitting). You may try sitting with a "donut" cushion to eliminate pressure on the tailbone, or limit sitting time in general.

Thoracic Spine

Although less common, some pregnant women experience pain in the thoracic spine during pregnancy. In large part, this is due to postural changes associated with distribution of weight gain, which cause an excess arch of the lower back, and excess rounding of the upper and mid-back. When the thoracic spine is rounded, the muscles and ligaments get overstretched. The muscles may spasm in response to this, which can propagate a cycle of pain.

During the third trimester as the baby grows, the abdominal organs get pushed up toward the chest and the rib cage gets crowded by the organs' upward displacement. The crowding within the abdominal cavity makes it more difficult to take a deep breath because the rib cage doesn't expand as well. As mentioned, the ribs connect to the thoracic spine, and with loss of rib expansion, there is loss of thoracic spine movement. The loss of mobility in this area can also contribute to pain. The most effective way to manage upper back pain is by posture correction, stretching, and deep breathing exercises.

CERVICAL SPINE

Neck pain can often be due to the stress of pregnancy and anticipating the birth of the baby. Many people, when under stress, unknowingly tighten and shrug up the shoulders. This can cause muscle spasm and decreased blood flow to the neck muscles, resulting in pain. It also alters the posture and alignment of the spine, and can place excess strain on the cervical spine joints. The postural change associated with pregnancy, where the upper back rounds excessively, contributes to the head jutting forward. This "forward head posture" puts strain on the muscles and joints, resulting in muscle spasm and pain. The best form of prevention and management is to relax, maintain good posture, and perform gentle stretching.

CHAPTER CONCLUSION

At this point, I hope you have a basic understanding of the anatomy of the spine and the physical changes that happen during pregnancy. The remainder of the book will focus on techniques for preventing and managing painful spinal conditions, with a large emphasis on exercise. The suggested program is one that can be used both during and after pregnancy, and I encourage you to be proactive throughout your life in preventing back pain by engaging in a regular exercise program.

~6~
Prevention and Management

Exercise Guidelines

Preventing back pain should be every woman's goal during pregnancy. The best strategy is to exercise appropriately, maintain good posture, and to move your body safely to minimize excess strain. If your attempts to prevent back problems are unsuccessful, or you are reading this book because you already have back pain, the following information should prove helpful in alleviating your symptoms.

The foundation for the back pain management program in this book is exercise. Although it may seem logical that if you are in pain you should rest and not undertake an exercise routine, gentle stretching and movement will often decrease muscle spasm and restore improved spinal alignment, resulting in decreased pain. If your pain is so severe that it prevents you from being able to perform any of the recommended exercises, you should contact your health care provider. Also, avoid taking any over the counter or prescription pain relievers and anti-inflammatories, which could be unsafe for your baby unless directed to do so by your physician.

You may experience some immediate pain relief from the following:

- **Ice/cold packs at the site of pain.** From my experience, I have found that cold packs used for 10–15 minutes every 1–2 hours as needed is effective in reducing muscle spasm and pain, likely due to their anti-inflammatory effect. Do not place an ice pack directly on the skin to avoid the risk of frostbite. Use a thin layer of clothing, towel, or pillowcase to protect your skin. If you experience acute onset of pain, ice/cold is recommended for at least the first 48 hours. If it seems to be helping, you may continue to use cold for several weeks as needed. I have had more success with ice/cold packs than heat with my clients, but different practitioners have different opinions and each woman is different.

- **Moist heat applied to muscles that are in spasm.** This helps increase circulation to the muscles, relieving pain. A moist warm towel or a sand filled moist hot pack can be applied to the site of pain for 10–15 minutes 2–3 times a day as needed. It is recommended to avoid heat application during the first 48 hours of a new injury, as it can increase swelling.

- **Warm bath, jacuzzi tub, or pool.** Water can be very soothing and help reduce muscle spasm and pain. Being immersed in water also minimizes the effects of gravity on the body, which is both relaxing and helpful in reducing pain. If you choose to go into a swimming pool, simply sitting, standing or walking in the water can be soothing. It is recommended that pregnant women avoid hot tubs and saunas, where extreme temperatures could cause problems including heat exhaustion, dizziness, and potential problems to the fetus if maternal core temperature rises.

- **Massage.** A partner, friend, or specialist can perform gentle massage to help relax muscles, increase circulation to them, and decrease pain. Some pregnant women find regular massage therapy to be beneficial for back pain management throughout their pregnancies. Be sure to consult with a therapist who specializes in prenatal massage.

From my experience, the benefits of cold, heat, warm baths, and massage are often temporary. If the underlying reason for pain is muscle imbalance, joint laxity, and poor posture, the above modalities will not correct the true problem. I strongly recommend you try the above with some combination of the exercises that will follow. (See the recommended daily program for acute pain in Chapter 12, which is a simple way to start moving.)

WHY EXERCISE?

By maximizing the flexibility, endurance, and strength of the muscles throughout your body, there will be fewer muscle imbalances, decreased stress on the loosening joints, and less dramatic changes in your posture, resulting in significantly less back pain. Exercise also helps to prevent excess weight gain, which contributes to strain on joints and increased postural dysfunction due to changes in your center of gravity.

AMERICAN COLLEGE OF OBSTETRICIANS AND GYNECOLOGISTS GUIDELINES

The American College of Obstetricians and Gynecologists (ACOG) established guidelines for safe exercise for pregnant women. The recommendations are general and designed to optimize the health of both mother and child, while minimizing risk to both. The recommendations are as follows.

Exercise Intensity

Many texts and physicians advise that pregnant women should exercise with a heart rate of less than 140 beats/minute. However in 1994, the ACOG updated their recommendations from the 140 heart rate limit. They now encourage women to listen to their bodies and respond to the way they feel during exercise, as there is less oxygen available to the exercising mother, with more oxygen providing nourishment to the baby. Exercising to fatigue, not exhaustion is considered safe and appropriate.

Another way to gauge the exercise intensity as being safe is with the "talk test." During the exercise routine, the woman should be able to talk without huffing and puffing. Although any exercise is better than none, it is important to note that a very slow leisurely walk around the block or at the mall should not be considered a conditioning exercise. The pace should be comfortable, yet somewhat challenging, in order for your body to benefit maximally.

Frequency of Exercise

It is recommended that the pregnant woman exercise at least three times per week, with sessions lasting 20-45 minutes.

Environmental Considerations

It is important to exercise in the proper environment. One concern, particularly during the first trimester, is a rise in core body temperature. This could result from exercise in extreme heat, which can be harmful to the baby. Be sure to exercise in a cool, well-ventilated area. If exercising outdoors in the summer, choose to do so in the morning or evening, when it tends to be cooler. Select clothing that absorbs perspiration and allows the skin to "breathe." Drink extra water to ensure adequate hydration.

Altitude is another factor to consider. Some studies have shown that women living in high altitudes when pregnant have decreased uterine blood flow. It is therefore recommended that women be careful to avoid exertion at high altitudes (greater than 8,250 feet) until at least 4–5 days exposure to adjust to the changed barometric pressure.

Physical Considerations

It is recommended that pregnant women avoid exercising supine (flat on their backs) after the first trimester. In the supine position, the weight of the growing baby can put pressure on the main blood vessels, resulting in decreased blood flow to the mother. If this occurs, the woman may feel lightheaded or dizzy and should turn to lie on her left side. The left sidelying position optimizes the circulation to both mother and child, and should alleviate any symptoms. If symptoms persist while laying on the left side, contact your health care provider immediately.

The type of exercise performed should be selected carefully. Any activity with a high risk for falling, such as skiing or horseback riding, should be avoided. Direct trauma to the abdomen from a fall can be harmful to the growing baby. In addition, there is an increased risk of spraining a joint due to the loosening of the ligaments. Any exercise that involves excess or repetitive spinal twisting or arching, such as tennis, golf, or gymnastics, should also be avoided due to the increased risk of a back injury. Activities that demand high level balance skills should be done with caution as the pregnant woman's balance declines due to changes in her center of gravity.

Pregnancy requires an additional 300 calories per day. The exercising pregnant woman should be more aware of selecting well-balanced meals and drinking an extra glass of water before and after exercise to maintain hydration. Fresh whole foods such as fruits, vegetables, nuts, and yogurt are health conscious choices for refueling the exercising body.

Choosing proper footwear is essential for comfort and safety during exercise and sports and is even more important when pregnant. As your ligaments become lax, the arches in the feet can drop slightly, causing many women to increase a whole shoe size while pregnant. Adding 25–35 pounds of weight on feet with falling arches can cause a great deal of discomfort. Fallen arches and other foot problems result in decreased shock absorption during weight bearing activities, and can result in increased stress on the ankles, knees, hips, and spine. A shoe with a good arch support will help maintain the normal structure of the foot, which decreases the risk of ankle, foot, knee, hip, and back strain.

Contraindications to Exercise

The ACOG recommends women not exercise in the presence of the following conditions:

- Pre-term Rupture of Membranes
- Pregnancy Induced Hypertension
- Incompetent Cervix
- Intrauterine Growth Retardation
- Persistent Bleeding in Second or Third Trimester
- Pre-Term Labor
- Multiple Gestation

If during a workout you experience any of the following symptoms, immediately stop the activity, and notify your health care provider:

- Pain
- Contractions
- Bleeding
- Shortness of Breath
- Palpitations or Heart Irregularities
- Rupture of Membranes or Vaginal Leakage
- Dizziness/Lightheadedness
- Blurred Vision/Seeing Spots

CHAPTER CONCLUSION

Based upon my education, professional and personal experience, and the ACOG guidelines, I have recommended a well-rounded exercise program for the pregnant woman consisting of cardiovascular, flexibility, and strength training. The combination of these types of exercise will help promote a good balance between muscle flexibility and strength, prevent excess weight gain, minimize postural changes, and thereby, decrease the risk of back pain. If you are already experiencing back or pelvic pain, the addition of a comprehensive exercise program can decrease the severity and/or intensity of pain or may eliminate pain entirely. It is important to keep in mind that not all types of back pain can be successfully treated with exercise alone. Be sure to discuss any problems with your health care provider, who may refer you to a specialist for individualized treatment.

~7~

Prevention and Management

Cardiovascular Conditioning

An activity that increases the body's heart rate for a sustained period of time is cardiovascular exercise. Walking, biking, swimming, jogging, elliptical training, stair climbing, and aerobics are all forms of cardiovascular exercise. The large muscle groups of the legs, trunk, and sometimes the arms work for a sustained period of time, during which blood is pumped faster through the muscles, heart, and lungs. The benefits of this type of exercise include improved muscle endurance, decreased risk of heart disease, decreased blood pressure, and increased energy level. (So don't try to use the "I'm pregnant and tired" excuse, because exercising will probably give you an energy boost.)

As a physical therapist, I recommend that my patients perform 20-45 minutes of cardiovascular exercise, 3-5 days a week. During pregnancy, women should exercise at a mild to moderate level, and not to the point of exhaustion. The activities I most often recommend to pregnant women follow:

- **Walking** is a good way to work the leg muscles with minimal impact and strain to the joints. Walking outdoors can be more interesting if you vary the routes and include small inclines some days to challenge yourself. Consider walking with a partner or friend to make the workout more fun and time pass quickly. Treadmill walking can be equally enjoyable, as you can vary speeds and incline levels, and it allows you to exercise in inclement weather. Avoid reading books or magazines on any gym fitness equipment as it tends to force you into poor posture, and increases the risk of losing your balance. Instead, listen to music to get you motivated and through the workout. Whether walking indoors or outdoors, keep the pace comfortable so you can still carry on a conversation.

- **Elliptical cross-training** is quite popular at most gyms and health clubs. The elliptical machine combines the motions of walking, climbing, and cycling, incorporating all the major muscles in the legs, with no impact at all, as your feet remain planted on foot pedals. Most elliptical trainers allow you to propel forward or backward, adjust the incline to vary the muscle groups worked, and adjust the intensity to an appropriate level for you. Some models also have swinging arms that you can push and pull to get an additional upper body workout (make sure you have good balance on the machine and feel confident prior to using the swinging arms). Because there is no impact, the elliptical is usually very comfortable and enjoyable during pregnancy. If you are unfamiliar with this equipment, ask a member of the health club staff to instruct you on safe use of the machine.

- **Bicycling** is another great no-impact activity that works the major muscle groups of the legs and improves total body endurance. During pregnancy, it is safer to use a stationary bike to avoid the risk of abdominal trauma due to falls on a regular bike. Early in pregnancy, some women find the recumbent bicycle to be more comfortable because it has a backrest to support the spine. As your baby and belly grow, it often becomes difficult to pedal due to the angle of the legs. The traditional stationary bike is as good as the recumbent and can generally be used throughout the entire pregnancy. Be careful not to slouch on the bike, as poor posture is a major contributor to back problems.

- **Swimming** is another excellent form of cardiovascular exercise. Water activities are relaxing and decrease the force of gravity acting on the spine, which can significantly improve back pain. If you are not a proficient swimmer but have back pain that prohibits you from participating in other forms of exercise, kicking while holding onto a kickboard, walking in waist deep water, or "pedaling on a noodle" are excellent alternatives. If like some women, you struggle with painful feet or varicose veins that weight-bearing exercises such as walking or the elliptical might aggravate, water exercise can be very soothing and allow you to remain fit and active.

Some fitness centers and hospitals offer pre-natal group exercise classes, which generally incorporate a combination of low

41

impact aerobics, strengthening, and stretching exercises designed specifically for the pregnant woman. Group exercise is a great place to meet other pregnant women and keeps some people more motivated to exercise. Make sure the instructor has training in pre-natal exercise so she or he knows what positions and exercises to avoid.

Running or jogging during pregnancy is usually not recommended since it is a high impact activity which can increase the risk of sprains or strains. If you are a seasoned runner, it is generally safe to continue jogging through the first trimester and even several weeks beyond. I recommend you transition to power walking as soon as you experience *any* difficulty or discomfort. If you were not previously a runner, pregnancy is not the time to start running but it is a good goal to set for yourself post-partum.

CHAPTER CONCLUSION

There are many types of cardiovascular exercise that are safe and enjoyable during pregnancy. It will help you remain fit and prevent or manage back pain in conjunction with the strength and flexibility exercises that are described in the subsequent chapters.

~8~

Prevention and Management

Strength Training

In addition to cardiovascular exercise, which optimizes muscle and cardiac endurance, it is important to maintain good muscle strength in order to maximize the stability around the spine and pelvis and to prepare your body for the work of labor and delivery. The pregnant woman benefits most from strengthening the abdominal, back, pelvic floor, buttock, and thigh muscles.

Some physicians advise women to stop all abdominal exercises after the first trimester to prevent a separation of the abdominal muscles. I recommend after 20 weeks gestation, women avoid performing crunches or sit-up type exercises, which require too much force for the stretching abdominals and can result in injury. Pelvic tilts, however, which work the abdominals, are safe and important to continue throughout pregnancy in order to prevent back pain and facilitate an easier delivery. Be sure to discuss with your health care provider their opinion regarding abdominal exercises after the first trimester.

It is recommended that the strengthening exercises be performed slowly and with control. The exercises can be performed for 10-20 total repetitions when beginning the program. As you become proficient, you can perform up to 30 repetitions. Breathe out during the exertion phase of the exercise, and inhale as you relax. Never hold your breath when strength training.

ABDOMINAL STRENGTHENING

The Pelvic Tilt

The pelvic tilt is a basic exercise that activates the lower abdominal muscles. Most people have difficulty isolating the lower abdominals and tend to do pelvic tilts incorrectly by using the buttock muscles. I will describe how to perform a pelvic tilt correctly and recommend you practice the technique until you have mastered it.

The simplest way to learn the pelvic tilt is to lay on your back with your knees bent, feet resting on the floor. Place your hand in the small of your back, and you will most likely notice a space between your back and the floor. Now try to flatten the lower part of the spine against the floor, so that you feel no space between your spine and the floor. What muscles do you feel working? If you feel your buttocks tightening, you are doing the exercise incorrectly. Relax the buttocks and place your hands just above the pubic bones along the lower part of the abdomen. Try to do the exercise again and feel the muscles under your hands along the lower abdomen tighten. Think about rotating the pelvis backwards, so the pubic bone tilts up towards your head and the spine presses into the floor. It is a small motion that is generated but an effective exercise. Hold the tilt for 3-5 seconds, and perform 2-3 sets of 10 repetitions. (If you still aren't sure if you are doing the pelvic tilt correctly, try increasing the arch in the lower back first, thereby increasing the space between the lower back and the floor. Now, reverse that motion and flatten your back. This back flattening is the direction you want to work on isolating.)

Pelvic Tilt in Supine

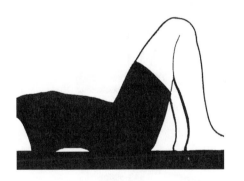 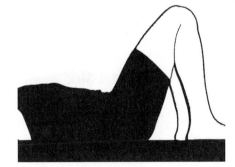

Start Position:
Note arch in lower back.

End Position:
Note absence of arch in lower back.

The pelvic tilt can be performed lying on your back, standing, in quadruped (on your hands and knees) and sitting. Each position provides an equally effective way to perform the pelvic tilt; if you master the sitting and standing variations, you can perform many pelvic tilts throughout your day, for example at work, in the car, or in line at the store. The pelvic tilt is a great means of toning the abdominals and relieving pressure on the lower back.

Pelvic Tilt in Quaruped

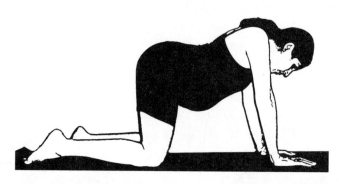

Start Position: Note arch in lower back.

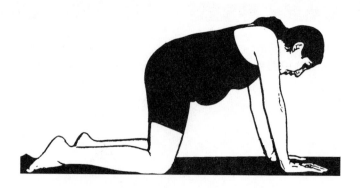

End Position: Note absence of arch in lower back.

Pelvic Tilt with Arms Overhead

Once you have mastered the pelvic tilt, there are advanced exercises that incorporate the tilt to provide an additional challenge to the abdominals. If you are still earlier than 20 weeks gestation, you could try these exercises. Hold a light weight (2-3 lbs) or a soup can in each hand while laying on your back. Do the pelvic tilt. Raise your arms up towards the ceiling at chest level, with your elbows straight. Slowly lower your arms back towards the ground, keeping the elbows straight. As you do this, your lower back will tend to arch off the floor. Keep tightening the abdominals so the lower back stays in contact with the floor. In other words, no movement of the pelvis or lower back should occur as you bring your arms

Pelvic Tilt with Arms Overhead

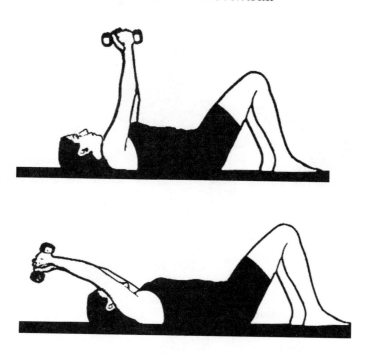

overhead, as long as you keep the abdominals working. Pause with the weight overhead for 1–2 seconds without letting your arms rest on the floor, and then return your arms to the start position. This exercise will engage the upper as well as lower abdominals.

Pelvic Tilt with Leg Marching

To challenge the lower abdominals more, try this variation of the pelvic tilt. While lying on your back, do a pelvic tilt. Without allowing the pelvis to shift, lift one leg off the floor, then slowly lower the leg, again without allowing the pelvis to shift. Alternate slowly lifting each leg, maintaining the pelvic tilt the entire time.

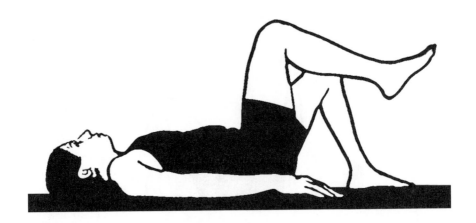

Pelvic Clocks

The pelvic clock exercise is another excellent means of isolating and strengthening the abdominal muscles. You may stand, sit, or lay on your back to perform the pelvic clocks. Start with your spine in its neutral position, and picture the ring of your pelvis as a clock, with 12 o'clock at your navel, 3 o'clock at your left hip, 6 o'clock at your pubic bone, and 9 o'clock at your right hip. Start by tilting your pelvis back towards 12 o'clock (this is the pelvic tilt you have been practicing). Without moving your legs or upper body, shift your pelvis towards the left to the 3 o'clock position. Slowly angle your pelvis down towards the 6 o'clock position, releasing the pelvic tilt and creating a very slight arch in the lower back. Now shift the pelvis to the right, or 9 o'clock position. Repeat this slowly and exaggerate each point on the pelvic clock. Try performing the exercise in both clockwise and counterclockwise directions.

BACK STRENGTHENING

Good strength of the upper and lower back is crucial for a pain free pregnancy. Due to postural changes, the back muscles tend to get weaker. When performing back strengthening exercises, avoid arching the lower back beyond a neutral position. Think about keeping a straight spine, with your abdominals contracting at the same time to counter the tendency to arch the back.

Quadruped Leg and Arm Lifts

The quadruped position is ideal for performing pelvic tilts as well as back strengthening. Start with a straight spine, and imagine a glass of water placed in the center of your lower back. Without letting your pelvis sway (or the imaginary glass of water spill) slowly lift one leg off the ground with the knee straight so you form a line from your toes to your head. Lower the leg, again maintaining a stable pelvis, and lift the opposite leg. This will strengthen the lower back, buttocks, and the hamstring in the back of the thigh.

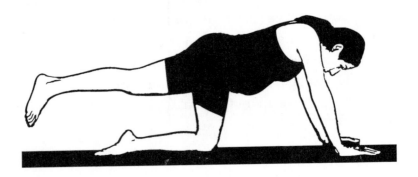

To target the upper back in this same position, try lifting one arm straight in front of you, again keeping the spine straight. Lower the arm slowly and repeat on the opposite side. This will strengthen the upper back and shoulder muscles.

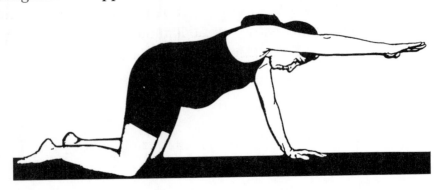

Once you feel comfortable with these two exercises and your balance in the quadruped position, you can combine them. Keeping the spine still, slowly lift the left leg and the right arm straight up. Slowly lower, and repeat with the right leg and left arm. This is a challenging and effective means of strengthening the spine. Do not perform this advanced version of the exercise if you are unable to maintain a stable pelvis.

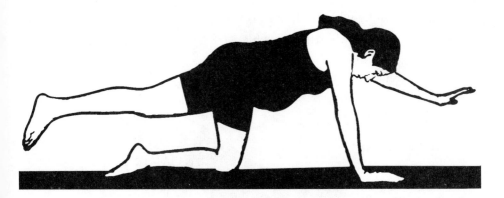

Bridging

This exercise is recommended up to 20 weeks of pregnancy. Lay on your back with your knees bent, feet resting on the floor. Tighten your abdominals and lift the buttocks off the floor by rolling up onto your shoulders. Keep your arms resting on the floor to provide added stability and balance. Avoid hyper extending (over-arching) the back, which should be in a straight line. Slowly lower down to the ground. This exercise strengthens the buttocks and lower back.

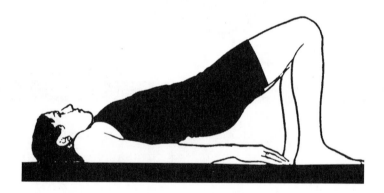

Row

Rowing can be done in various ways, but the basic concept is the same. Keeping your lower back in a neutral position, pull the arms back with elbows bent, and squeeze your shoulder blades together. Slowly return to the starting position. This exercise will strengthen the muscles of the upper back, shoulders, and arms.

You can do a bent over row with three to eight pound free weights. Rest one knee on a chair, lean forward at the hips, keep your back straight, and use one hand on the backrest of the chair

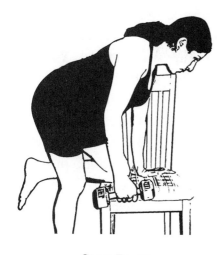

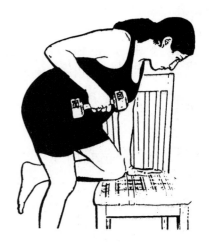

Start Position   *End Position*

to help with your balance. Hold the weight in your free hand with your elbow straight, pull your arm back, and squeeze your shoulder blade towards the center of your spine. If you do not lean forward adequately, you will not likely feel the upper back muscles getting a workout. Look in a mirror to confirm your position.

PELVIC FLOOR STRENGTHENING: KEGEL EXERCISES

The pelvic floor muscles are key for supporting the bladder, bowel, uterus, and weight of your growing baby. These are the muscles through which the baby passes during a vaginal birth. In order for the pelvic floor to stretch to accommodate the baby, the muscles must be strong and pliable. A strong pelvic floor also helps prevent incontinence (leakage of urine) late in pregnancy and post-partum. Kegel exercises can be difficult to learn, but practice often, and you will become proficient at performing them.

To exercise the pelvic floor muscles, try to envision pulling the muscles of the saddle area up and in towards your baby. You should not feel your buttocks, thighs, or abdominals tightening as you do this. One of the simplest ways to learn to contract the pelvic floor is to stop the flow of urine while you are on the toilet. You can try this technique to verify which muscles to isolate, but avoid doing this often, as it can cause urinary tract infections.

When you first learn the Kegel exercise, hold the contraction for 3-5 seconds then relax. Repeat this 10 times, 2–3 sets. After you master the standard Kegel, try the "elevator" variation: pull the pelvic floor muscles up a little, then a little higher, then a little higher, like an elevator climbing up 3–4 levels. Slowly release down little by little as you relax the muscles again.

As previously mentioned, the Kegel exercise can help to facilitate a smooth delivery. When the pelvic floor is strong it is better able to help push the baby out; it also can respond better to the demands to stretch and expand to allow the passage of the baby. Equally important is its role in preventing incontinence in later pregnancy and postpartum. Late in pregnancy as your baby grows, more weight is being pressed down on the pelvic floor, which can weaken it. After a vaginal delivery, these muscles are further stretched to the point where simply laughing, coughing, or sneezing can cause you to leak small or large amounts of urine. This can be prevented by continuing Kegel exercises post-partum. Be sure to also discuss any problems you experience with incontinence with your health care provider.

SQUATS

Squatting helps strengthen the muscles in the thighs, buttocks, low back, abdominals, and pelvic floor. Further, the squatting position is one used during labor as it opens the pelvic outlet optimally in order to facilitate the baby moving further down. Practicing squats and attaining good strength in these muscles not only helps manage back pain, but will also be helpful for your labor and delivery. There are four variations of the squat that will be described here. In the first three types of squats do not let your knees move past your toes, as it can cause undue strain to the knee joints, and only squat as low as is comfortable for you.

The Wall Squat

Wall squatting is an easy way to practice squatting with good form. Stand with your head, shoulders, and back against a wall with your feet shoulders width apart, about 1-2 feet away from the wall. Do a pelvic tilt, so the lower back presses into the wall. Squat as if you were going to sit down, and maintain contact between your back and the wall. Pause in the lowest squat position that is comfortable with the knees approaching a 90-degree angle. Come back up slowly, keeping your back and buttocks in contact with the wall.

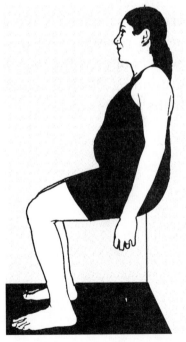

Note that knees do not move past the toes.

The Traditional Squat

In traditional squats, it is important to watch in a mirror as you
perform them, to ensure safe
form and avoid injury to the
back or knees. Start in an
upright position with your feet
shoulder width apart. With the
abdominals contracted, squat
down as if you are going to sit in
a chair that is directly behind
you. (It may be helpful to actual-
ly place a chair behind you to
ensure you move in the correct
form.) Your spine should be in a
neutral position, and the knees
should not pass the toes. Return
to standing slowly, squeezing the
thighs and buttocks.

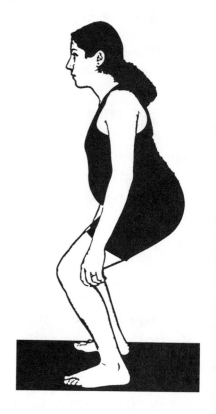

The Ballet Squat

Ballet, or adductor, squats work the muscles of the inner thighs. These muscles are pelvic stabilizers and important for the health of your spine. Stand with your feet wider than shoulders width apart with your toes pointing out. Squat down like a ballerina's plié, again, without letting the knees go past the toes. Squeeze the inner thigh muscles as you return to standing.

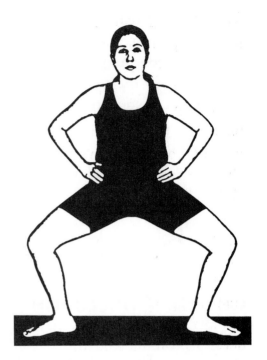

The Deep Squat

Deep squatting helps improve the flexibility of the inner thighs, which need to be limber in order to assume many of the commonly used labor positions. It also helps strengthen the thighs, back, and pelvic floor. Deep squats can be very challenging, especially in later pregnancy. If you do not have good flexibility in the lower back and legs, it will be difficult to perform correctly; therefore, only try these if you experience no discomfort and can maintain good alignment. *If you have a history of knee problems, do not perform this exercise.*

With your feet slightly wider than shoulders width apart and feet turned outward, squat all the way down to the ground, keeping your heels flat and spine straight. Use your hands to press your knees slightly apart. Try to sustain the deep squat for 15-20 seconds, and gradually increase the time to 30 seconds. If you become proficient at this, you can also do your Kegel exercises in this position for an additional challenge.

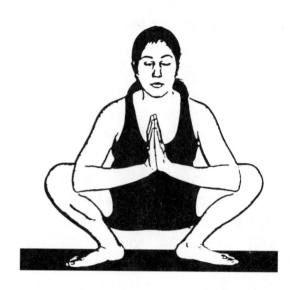

CHAPTER CONCLUSION

Although there are numerous other strengthening exercises that are safe to perform during pregnancy, those listed above are most beneficial in preventing and managing back pain, as well as preparing your body for the baby's delivery. In addition to cardiovascular and strength training, stretching is key for a healthy spine and easier delivery.

~9~

Prevention and Management

Stretching

Many patients I work with are faithful when it comes to walking and doing strength training, but a lot of them skip the stretching due to time constraints and the feeling that it is somehow less important. Stretching is at least as important as cardiovascular and strength training for injury prevention and rehabilitation. It is better to do a shorter cardiovascular and strengthening workout in order to save time for stretching, than to sacrifice this crucial component of the exercise program.

The goal of improving flexibility is for the muscles to achieve a new lengthened resting position. When muscles are flexible, or lengthened, they do not put excess tension on joints, thereby decreasing the likelihood of pain and injury. In order to improve flexibility, it is recommended that stretches be performed after you are warmed up from a workout or warm shower. Hold the stretches (never bounce) for 20-30 seconds, and repeat 3 times. In order for the muscles to learn their new lengthened position, you should stretch at least twice a day. Stretching once a day is necessary to maintain the improved muscle length. In other words, once you have achieved better flexibility, you should stretch once a day to maintain it. It may seem overwhelming to think you have to find time to stretch once or twice a day, however a few minutes of stretching is well worth your time and effort. You can try performing the stretches throughout the day so it will seem less daunting.

Avoid stretching to the point of pain; you should feel a strong pulling sensation that may be uncomfortable, but should not be painful. For many of the muscle stretches that are suggested, there are various positions that will provide appropriate stretching. During the first trimester, the supine (laying flat on your back) exercises are safe. After 20 weeks, it is recommended that you perform the seated or standing variations of the stretches.

THE BACK STRETCH

The back muscles tend to get tight from the postural changes that occur during pregnancy. This stretch elongates the muscles along the entire spine to give a stretch to the muscles that travel from the neck to the lower back. It also helps reverse the excess arch that tends to be present in the lower back during pregnancy.

Start on your hands and knees, with your legs wide apart. Place a small pillow under you to give support to your abdomen. Sit back on your knees and stretch your arms forward to feel a stretch along the spine.

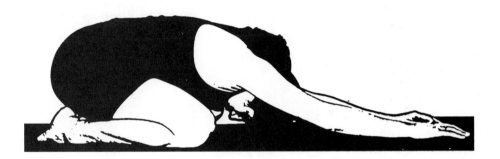

THE ADDUCTOR STRETCH

The adductors, or inner thigh muscles, connect from the thighs to the pelvis and provide stability to the pelvis and lower back. The adductors need to be flexible in order to assume various labor and delivery positions, such as squatting, semi-reclined with feet in stirrups, or side lying. The stretch can be performed either sitting or standing. *Do not perform these stretches if you have a separated pubic symphysis as it can aggravate the condition.*

Variation #1: Standing

Standing with your spine in neutral and your feet about three to four feet apart turn your toes out and bend one knee as you shift your weight onto the bent leg. You should feel a stretch on the inner thigh of the leg that is straight.

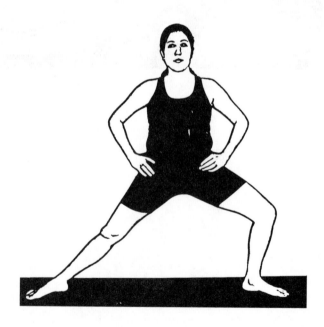

Variation #2: Sitting Butterfly

There are two seated variations to the adductor stretch: the butterfly and "V" stretches. The butterfly stretch requires that you sit on the floor with your spine straight and both knees bent with the soles of your feet touching each other. Try to press the knees down towards the ground, keeping the spine straight.

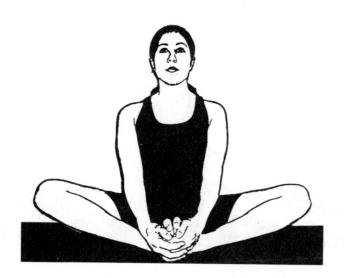

Variation #3: Sitting "V"

For the "V" stretch, sit on the floor with your back straight. Extend your legs in front of you with your hips wide apart and knees straight. Slightly lean forward from the hips, keeping the spine straight to increase the stretch. This may be difficult if you have tightness in the hamstrings or lower back. If you notice your lower back rounding or that you are unable to sit straight, choose the standing or butterfly stretch to avoid excess strain to the lower back.

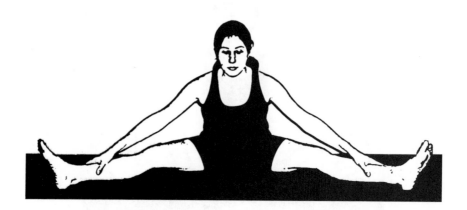

THE PIRIFORMIS STRETCH

The piriformis muscle, located deep within the buttock region, connects from the sacrum to the hip. The sciatic nerve travels between fibers of the piriformis muscle, and tightness in the piriformis can be a cause of sciatica. This muscle needs to be flexible in order to prevent irritation to the sciatic nerve, allow the sacrum to maintain good movement and alignment, and allow the hips to spread for labor and delivery. Stretching can be done supine, sitting, or in a modified-standing position.

Variation #1: Supine

Lay on your back with your knees bent and cross the right foot over the left knee. Hold behind the left leg and pull both legs in towards the chest. You will feel a stretch along the right buttocks. Repeat on the opposite side.

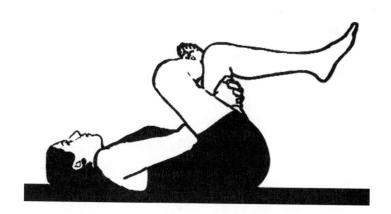

Variation #2: Sitting

Sit with your back straight and cross the left foot over the right knee. Gently press the left knee towards the floor. To increase the stretch, bend forward from the hips. Repeat on the opposite side.

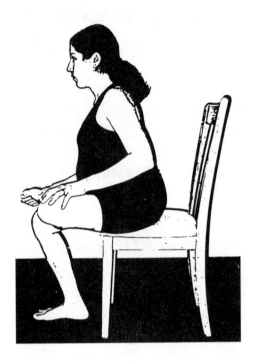

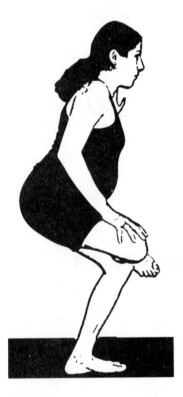

Variation #3: Modified Standing

Stand and cross the right foot over the left knee. Hold onto a wall or a chair and gently squat down to feel a stretch in the right buttock area. Repeat on the opposite side.

THE HAMSTRING STRETCH

The hamstrings are the large group of muscles that run along the back of the thigh from the pelvis to the knee. Hamstring tightness can result in misalignment in the pelvis and excess strain on the lower back. The majority of people with back pain (pregnant or not) have tight hamstrings, often due to poor posture.

Variation #1: Supine

Lay on your back with both legs flat on the ground, toes pointing up towards the ceiling. Using a belt or a towel around one foot, pull that leg up towards a 90 degree angle at the hip, keeping your knee as straight as possible. Keep your head and neck relaxed. Also keep the opposite leg pressed against the floor. If you are unable to do the stretch without feeling lower back or hip strain, keep the opposite leg bent. As you gain flexibility, again try to straighten that leg.

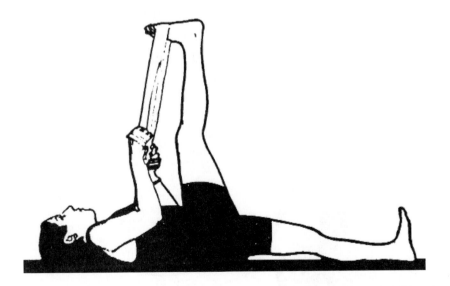

Variation #2: Standing

Facing a chair or a step, place one foot up on it, keeping both hips and feet facing forward. Keeping your back straight, lean forward from the hips to increase the stretch. If you are unable to keep your back straight or your knees start to bend, the chair or step is likely too high for your flexibility level. Try a lower surface.

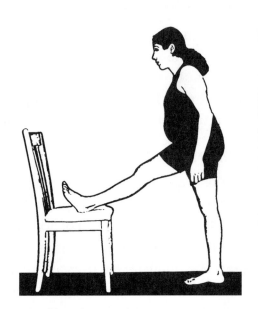

Variation #3: Sitting

Sit on the floor with your back straight and your legs extended straight in front of you. Reach for your toes by bending forward from the hips, keeping your back straight. You may also use a towel or a belt around your feet to assist in this stretch.

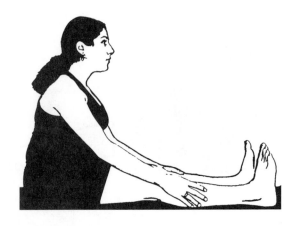

THE PSOAS AND QUADRICEPS STRETCH

The psoas (pronounced "so-as") muscle is situated in the front of the pelvis, traveling from the hip to the vertebrae in the lower back. The quadriceps are the large thigh muscles in the front of the leg. When tight, these muscles pull the pelvis forward, and place excess stress on the lower back. The psoas and quadriceps can be stretched in either standing or kneeling positions. When stretching these muscles in any position, avoid over-arching the lower back.

Variation #1: Standing

Stand with your spine straight, bend your knee, and grab onto your ankle. Bring your heel up towards the buttocks to feel a stretch in the front of the thigh. Check your form to make sure you are not pulling your leg out to the side. Your knees should stay together. If you are unable to comfortably grab onto your ankle or keep your knees together, you should perform the next variation of this stretch using a chair to prevent undue strain to your knees or spine.

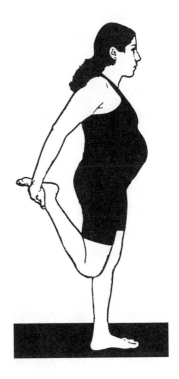

Variation #2 Standing Chair Stretch

Stand holding onto a wall or counter with a chair behind you. Place your foot on the seat of the chair, and gently squat down to feel a stretch in the front of the hip and thigh. Be sure to keep both knees toward the midline of your body, and maintain a neutral spine. If you do not feel a stretch, you may need to place your foot on a higher surface, such as the armrest of a chair.

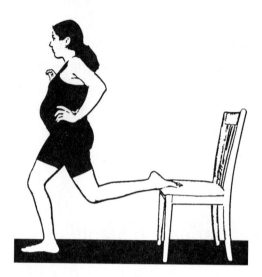

Variation #3: Kneeling

Kneel on the floor, with one leg in front of you with the hip and knee at 90-degree angles. Do a pelvic tilt, and then gently lean forward to feel a stretch along the front of the hip and thigh of the leg that is positioned behind you. This stretch will be felt higher up towards the hip, as it isolates the psoas, or hip flexor muscle, more so than the quadriceps.

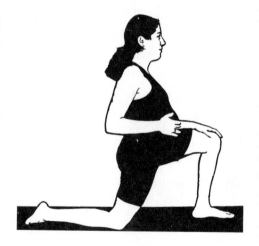

THE SIDE WAIST AND HIP STRETCH

The muscles on the sides of the waist encompass the oblique abdominal muscles, back muscles, and the muscles that connect along the ribs. These muscles all tend to be tight due to postural changes associated with pregnancy. The outer hip muscles, or iliotibial band and hip abductors, can also become tight and place strain on the pelvis. This stretch opens the side waist and hip areas, to decrease discomfort and improve spinal mobility.

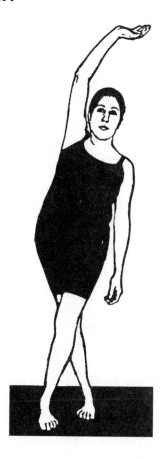

Stand with your spine in its neutral position. Bring your right leg behind the left, keeping your toes pointing forward. Stick your right hip out towards the right wall as you gently reach your right arm overhead and lean your torso towards the left. You will feel a stretch along the right waist and outer hip. Repeat the stretch on the left side.

THE PECTORAL STRETCH

The pectorals are muscles in the front of the chest and shoulders that often become tight due to postural changes associated with pregnancy. Tightness in this muscle group causes the thoracic spine and shoulders to be excessively rounded. Stretching this muscle group will relieve upper back and neck discomfort, improve posture, and decrease shoulder strain.

Standing Variation #1

Stand with each hand at shoulder level with your hands on the walls in a corner or on the sides of a doorframe. Keeping your head up and your back straight, lean forward to feel a stretch in the front of your shoulders and chest.

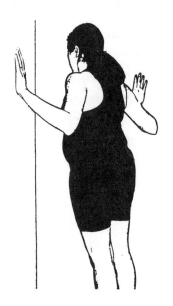

Standing Variation #2

Stand with your head upright and your back straight. Clasp your hands behind your back, and without leaning your shoulders forward, gently stretch your arms back and up to feel a stretch in the front of your shoulders and arms.

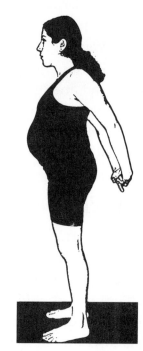

THE THORACIC SPINE STRETCH

Pain in the upper back between the shoulder blades is a common complaint during pregnancy due to the postural changes and decreased rib excursion late in pregnancy as your baby grows. Doing a gentle stretch combined with deep breaths can help improve flexibility in this region.

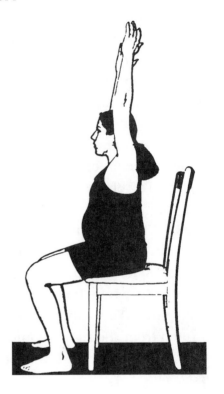

Sitting upright in a chair, do a pelvic tilt to keep your lower back stabilized. With your arms straight, reach overhead as high as you can while you take a deep breath in. Gently push your chest forward to arch the upper back, without allowing the lower back to arch. Slowly lower your arms back down as you exhale. Hold the stretch for 3–5 seconds and repeat this 10 times. Although not pictured, this stretch can also be performed standing.

THE NECK STRETCH

The muscles along the sides of the neck, the upper trapezius, are a common area of tightness and tension in many individuals, pregnant or not. Due to postural changes and increased stress during pregnancy, you may notice discomfort in the neck region. To relieve this, try bringing your right arm behind your back. While keeping your back straight, tilt your head gently to the left side. Be sure you do not allow your whole body to lean to the side. You should feel a stretch from the right shoulder to the neck. Repeat on the opposite side.

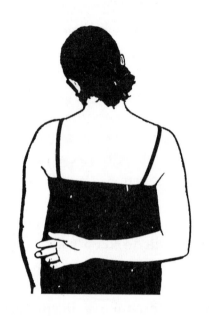

CHAPTER CONCLUSION

Stretching is one key component to a healthy, pain-free spine during pregnancy, along with cardiovascular and strength training. Stretching also helps improve your posture by decreasing muscle tightness that might cause you to slouch or move out of your ideal alignment. Postural awareness in terms of how you use and move your body during everyday tasks is another key factor in managing and preventing back pain, and is discussed in the next chapter.

~10~
Prevention and Management

Posture and Body Mechanics

Good posture is something few people consistently demonstrate. If you look at people around you, chances are many of them will be slouching or standing with their weight shifted onto one leg or leaning up against something. Even as a physical therapist, I find myself straightening up before explaining to new patients how their poor posture is a likely cause of their pain. The fact is that good posture, or what has previously been described as neutral spine posture, can be hard to maintain. It requires a good balance between muscle strength and flexibility, and more importantly, a keen sense of awareness of how you move and position your body during activities. During pregnancy, it is even more crucial to be aware of your posture and body mechanics (how you use or move your body to accomplish a task) due to joint laxity and an increased risk of strain to the spine.

The basic concept is to attempt to maintain a neutral spine posture no matter what you do. In other words, keep the natural curves of the spine present with whatever activity you are doing. Some people think it only pertains to strenuous activities, such as lifting something very heavy, but in fact it should be applied to tasks as simple as brushing your teeth. This section will illustrate the use of good posture and body mechanics in everyday situations.

SLEEP POSITIONS

A challenge for most pregnant women is finding a comfortable position that allows an uninterrupted night's sleep. The most common recommended sleep position during pregnancy is in a side lying position, preferably on the left side, as there is optimal blood flow to both the mother and baby. Positioning with pillows is the key to keeping your spine neutral in bed. If you toss and turn, the pillows may not be there when you wake up, but at least start out the night with good alignment to increase your odds of a better sleep position. Your head pillow should be providing your neck with a supportive, yet comfortable cushion. Your head should not be tilted up (the pillow is too high or firm, or you use too many pillows) or slanting down (the pillow is too low or soft). You may want to try a pillow designed for side sleeping or a specially designed cervical pillow that has a contoured shape to support the space between your head and shoulders.

When you lay on your side, your top leg will drop down to rest on your bottom leg, placing strain on the pelvis. Sleeping with a pillow between your knees keeps the legs separated in order to allow the pelvis to remain in its neutral position. You may need two pillows to accomplish this. As your baby grows, so will your belly, which can make lying on your side uncomfortable. Some women find that placing a small pillow under the abdomen gives additional support and comfort to the growing weight of the baby.

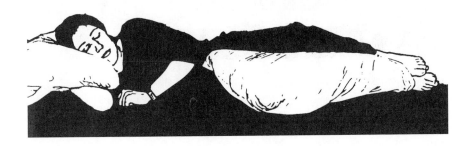

During the last month of pregnancy, some women find it difficult to breathe as the baby displaces the abdominal organs up towards the ribcage, limiting the expansion capacity of the lungs. This is often worse with exertion or when lying down. If you experience difficulty breathing, you may be more comfortable in a semi-reclined sleep position, which will also require multiple pillows behind your head and back to prop you up, and 1–2 pillows under your knees to decrease strain on the lower back. Again, don't worry if you wake up in a different position than you intended.

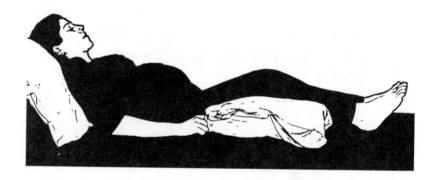

GETTING IN AND OUT OF BED

There is a right and a wrong way to get out of bed, whether or not you are pregnant. If you are on your back, roll onto your side with your knees bent. If you are a side sleeper, you will already be in this position. Bring your legs over the side of the bed as you simultaneously push your torso up to a sitting position. The incorrect method is to transition from supine (flat on your back) to a long sitting position (sitting with legs straight in front of you). This movement requires significant abdominal strength and places strain on the lower back. During pregnancy when the abdominals are stretched and weaker, they are less efficient and the chances of injury are even greater.

Once seated, it is a good idea to wait a minute prior to standing so you don't get dizzy.

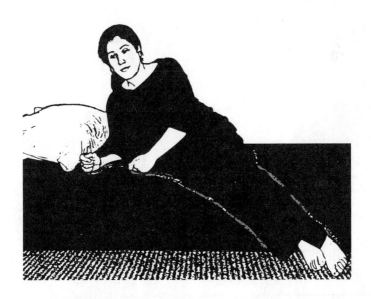

SITTING POSTURE

The key to good sitting posture is to keep the spine well supported in order to maintain its natural curves. Without good support, the postural muscles have to work continuously to keep the spine neutral, which can be difficult and fatiguing. Sit with your buttocks and lower back all the way to the back of the chair. If the chair is too deep for you (many couches and oversized chairs are too deep for shorter women), place a pillow behind your back to prop you forward. Your hips and knees should be positioned at approximately 90-degree angles, and your feet should rest comfortably on the floor. If the chair is too high, place a stool at your feet. If using an office chair, adjust the back so the lumbar support lines up with your lower back. Crossing your legs when seated is not recommended as it can hinder circulation and aggravate varicose veins.

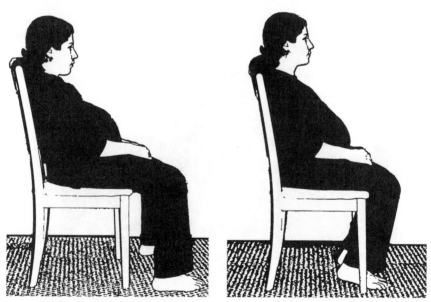

Don't slouch. Sit back in the chair for better posture.

Transition from Sitting to Standing

If moving from a seated to standing position is painful, here is a technique that might make the task easier. Keeping your spine straight, scoot to the front of the chair. Tighten your abdominals, push off with your hands, and stand up keeping your back straight. Avoid bending forward as you stand, as this can place stress on the spine.

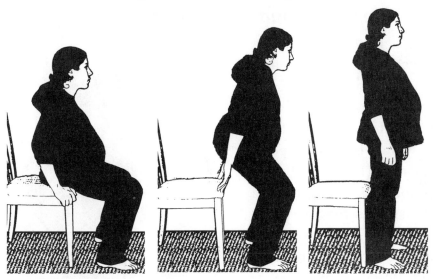

Standing Posture

When standing, many people tend to lean backward, shift their weight onto one leg, or slouch. All of these positions bring the spine out of its neutral alignment and increase the risk of injury. If you are standing for a prolonged period and are unable to sit, try leaning your entire back against a wall, with your feet about 12 inches away from the wall. You can also try placing one foot up on a step or stool, alternating legs every few minutes. These techniques will give your postural muscles a rest, while maintaining the natural curves of the spine.

ACTIVITIES OF DAILY LIVING

As you read this section, it may seem ludicrous to think about how you brush your teeth or vacuum. However, I can't count the number of patients who have experienced pain during the various activities below and have noticed significant improvement when they have changed their habits.

Brushing Teeth and Washing Face

Basic hygiene, such as brushing your teeth and washing your face, is something everyone does without thinking about how their bodies are positioned. The majority of people bend slightly over the sink as they do these activities, and even this minor bending can place additional stress on a painful or weak spine. Try instead to squat down slightly, resting your forearms on the sink or countertop. You can also place one foot on a stool or

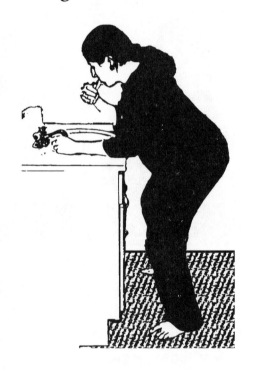

inside the base of the sink cabinet. This will allow you to maintain a neutral spine alignment, and take some pressure off your back.

Vacuuming

The chore of vacuuming can be taxing on the spine if done without care. Instead of reaching, leaning and twisting while standing in one spot, move with the vacuum cleaner keeping it close to you, and work in one small area at a time. If you catch sight of dirt off to your side, turn to face it with the vacuum 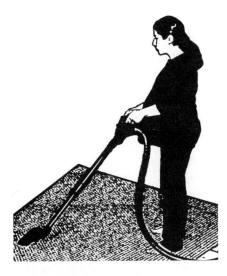 cleaner. It may seem to take a little longer, but if it prevents you from experiencing pain, it will be well worth it.

Getting Shoes On

The challenge of reaching past your belly to put on socks and shoes can be a daunting task. In terms of posture, it is ideal to sit when putting on your shoes and socks. Bring one leg up and cross it over the opposite leg, keeping your back straight.

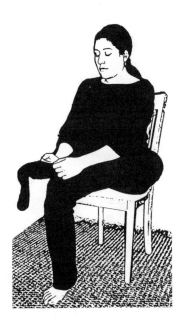

Lifting

There are five major points to consider when lifting:

- **Lift with your legs, not your back.** Keep your back straight and squat down to pick up the object, however heavy or light.

- **Keep it close to you.** When you keep the object you are lifting close to your body, your spine experiences less strain.

- **Don't twist.** If you are moving something from one place to another, turn your whole body as opposed to turning at the waist. This eliminates strain from rotating with a load.

- **Know how heavy the object is before attempting to lift it.**

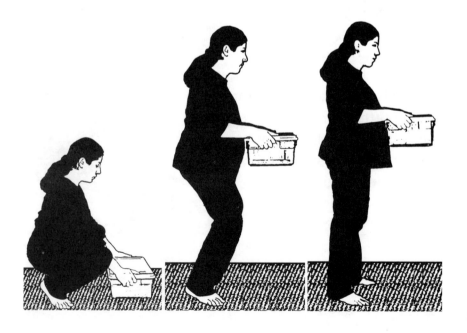

- **Get help lifting any heavy or awkward objects.** If two or more people are working together, be sure to plan the lift and destination of the object. Have one person in charge to direct the lift.

Stretch Breaks

With awareness and effort, great improvements can be made in terms of an individual's posture and body mechanics. Inevitably, poor postural habits will creep into your everyday life at some point. For example, while typing now, I feel myself having to straighten up in my chair and stretch to reverse my slouched posture. It feels better to stretch and undo the stress on the spine. A key to decreasing postural strain is to frequently change your position or activity. The shorter period of time spent performing the same task, the less likely your muscles will fatigue, and the less chance you have for injury. Try to change your position at least every half-hour and take stretch breaks. If you easily lose track of time, you may find it helpful to set an alarm to remind you to change your position.

There are two postural exercises I recommend. The purpose of these stretches is to "undo," or reverse the tendency for the spine to be slouched. I recommend you perform these once or twice daily. If you have a job that requires you to be in any one position for long periods of time, it is recommended you perform these exercises several times throughout the workday.

Wall Posture Exercise

Stand with your head, shoulders and back against a wall with your feet shoulders width apart, about 1–2 feet from the wall. Bring your arms out to your sides with your palms facing away from the wall. Do a pelvic tilt to press the lower back into the wall. Press your thoracic spine and shoulders against the wall without letting your lower back move away from the wall. Next, press the back of your head back into the wall, without tilting your chin up or down. You should feel a stretch along the entire spine if you do this correctly. Hold the stretch for 15–20 seconds, and repeat 3 times.

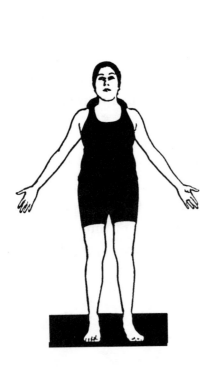
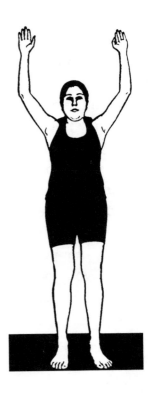

Once this exercise gets easier, raise your arms higher overhead to challenge yourself. You can also bring your feet closer to the wall. The wall posture exercise not only stretches the postural muscles, it also strengthens them as you try to maintain the position.

Chin Tuck

The chin tuck exercise helps to reverse the tendency most people have to allow the head jut forward. The goal is to bring the head back into alignment over the spine, so the ears line up over the shoulders. It is best to practice this exercise in front of a mirror to assure that your form is correct. Stand with your spine straight. Pull your head straight back, without tilting your chin up or down, and try to make a double chin. Your jaw should remain relaxed. You will feel the muscles along the back of the neck stretching.

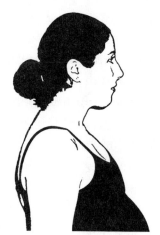

Start Position: Note that due to postural changes at late pregnancy, head is in a forward position.

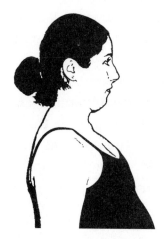

End Position: Pull head straight back to align ear over shoulder.

Hold the chin tuck for 3–5 seconds and relax to the start position. Repeat 10 times. The chin tuck is an easy exercise to do at stop lights or when stopped in traffic (never when driving), as many people tend to sit slouched and tense up when dealing with the stress of their commute. The chin tuck will help improve posture and decrease muscle tension.

CHAPTER CONCLUSION

Gaining awareness of your posture and body mechanics is a process that takes some time. I always tell my patients that if they catch themselves doing a task incorrectly, they've mastered the hardest part of the process. Each time you correct yourself, you eliminate a small degree of strain to the spine. Just as the more you do incorrectly, the more likely you are to feel pain, the more you do with good posture and body mechanics, the less likely you are to feel pain.

The previous information regarding posture and body mechanics completes the program for prenatal back pain management. The combination of cardiovascular conditioning, strengthening, stretching, and postural improvement will help optimize the balance between strength and flexibility in the spine as your body changes. Achieving this balance is essential for preventing and managing back pain both during pregnancy and post-partum.

~11~

Management of Post-Partum Back Pain

It is not uncommon to experience post-partum back pain. Some women who sailed through pregnancy without any back pain can be disappointed to be plagued with post-partum pain. The process of childbirth is a marathon of sorts, often requiring great effort, determination, and strength. Just as running 26 plus miles would likely leave you feeling sore, so can childbirth. For many, the soreness is due to muscle strain, and will resolve spontaneously within days. If you had an epidural, you may experience pain at the insertion site. For others, post-partum back or pelvic pain can be a lingering problem. I will briefly explain some causes of post-partum back and pelvic pain, and describe management techniques.

YOUR HEALING BODY

Over a period of nine months your body gradually changed as your baby developed. The big day came, your baby is now here, but whose body is staring back at you in the mirror? You may find yourself still looking seven months pregnant, but do not worry. Extra fluid, distension of the bowels, your enlarged uterus, and yes, some weight gain, are the causative factors. Although in today's society women are expected to be home and functioning just days after birth, the body needs time to heal and return to its pre-pregnancy state.

The joints throughout the body remain lax after birth due to continued hormonal changes, and the abdominal and pelvic floor muscles that have been stretched out of shape need to shrink back down and regain strength to provide spinal and pelvic stability. Weakness in the muscles can result in excess mobility in the lower back and pelvis, which can create inflammation and pain. The spine and pelvis should be considered unstable until the hormones return to pre-pregnancy levels and the abdominal and pelvic floor muscles regain their strength.

Due to an instant weight loss of about 10–12 pounds (baby, amniotic fluid, placenta, and blood), your center of gravity, which has gradually shifted during pregnancy, experiences a sudden shift back again. This will affect posture and can result in lower back pain. The use of good posture and body mechanics will help minimize the effects of the sudden weight change.

The type of delivery you experience will also affect how you feel and the type of recovery you can expect. The differences between a vaginal and cesarean delivery seem obvious, but there are physio-logical factors to consider in terms of causes of low back pain and consequently how to best manage it.

VAGINAL DELIVERY

In a vaginal delivery, the pelvic outlet widens and the pelvic floor muscles stretch significantly, allowing the baby to pass through the otherwise small vaginal opening. The pelvic joints can get forced out of alignment as the baby descends, in order to create more space. For example, often in the case of a baby with a large head where a long period of time is spent pushing, the pubic symphysis can shear, where one side moves forward with respect to the opposite side. A misalignment of the pelvis will stress ligaments and muscles surrounding the affected joints and result in pain. Professional treatment by a physical therapist (preferably one with experience in muscle energy techniques and pre-natal/post-partum care) or other specialist is recommended to correct a suspected post-partum skeletal alignment problem.

The pelvic floor muscles stretch as the baby exits the vagina; and as with any overstretched muscle, it can become painful and inflamed. There will often be small micro tears within the pelvic floor, with some tears significant enough to require stitches. Your obstetrician may have chosen to perform an episiotomy, where an incision was made in the pelvic floor muscles to allow a greater space for the baby to pass through and to avoid severe tearing of these muscles. In any of these circumstances, the tissue of the pelvic floor takes 6–8 weeks to fully heal. There will be associated scar tissue and weakness in these muscles as a result of the trauma, and if not addressed, can result in chronic pelvic pain and dysfunction. Gently massaging the pelvic floor muscles (begin 6 weeks post-partum after getting approval from your health care provider) will help break up any scar tissue that may have formed and help re-align the muscle fibers.

CESAREAN SECTION

If you delivered by cesarean section, your pelvic floor may have been spared some trauma, but your abdominal incision will slow your recovery. Not only were your abdominals stretched out over your bulging belly for the last several months, but also they've been cut through to deliver your baby. The result is significant weakness in the abdominals. As previously discussed, weak abdominals are a precursor to back pain, especially in an unstable spine.

Your incision will take a full 6-8 weeks to heal, and once healed scar tissue will have formed at the site of the incision. The presence of scar tissue in the abdominals will limit how well they will contract. Once fully healed, it is important that you perform gentle scar massage perpendicular to the incision in order to break up any scar tissue. The incision will initially feel tender and lumpy. As the scar tissue dissipates, it will feel less sensitive and suppler.

MANAGING POST-PARTUM BACK PAIN

Unfortunately, your pregnant body does not return to its pre-pregnancy state overnight. It takes hard work to get back to good physical condition, but returning to your normal weight and restoring the strength of the abdominal, pelvic floor and back muscles will be key to managing post-partum back pain. It is generally recommended that following childbirth, the mother wait six weeks to return to exercise. In part, I agree with this, given that the body is healing and the unstable pelvis and spine are vulnerable to injury. Strenuous exercise, such as jogging, biking, and heavy weight lifting should be avoided early post-partum. However, it is safe to engage in a program of walking, isometric exercises, and gentle stretching as soon as you feel up to it. These early exercises will help get you back into shape, facilitate the weight loss process, help manage back pain, and prepare you for returning to your normal activity level.

WALKING

It is safe to begin walking for exercise when you arrive home; however, do not expect to start out with a power walk. Your body is healing and will respond best to a gradually implemented walking program. I remember after having my son, going out for a walk. I moved at a snail's pace, and probably ventured less than a quarter mile in 20 minutes. Each successive day, I was able to go a little further and a little faster. To help regain your endurance, it may be easier to do a few very short walks each day until you can tolerate a greater distance. You will need to save energy to care for your newborn and allow your body to recuperate. If you have a winter baby in a cold or snowy climate and you can't walk outside, start with short walks around your home and graduate to walking indoors at a mall or on a treadmill. If you start out on a treadmill, use caution and keep the speed very slow.

It is important in this early post-partum phase to be receptive to how you feel and adjust your walking accordingly. If a ten minute walk leaves you feeling winded and fatigued, you've either walked too far or at too rapid a pace. You should also monitor the flow of lochia (bloody discharge that is normal following pregnancy) as you begin exercising. If you notice that the flow becomes heavier, your body is telling you to slow down.

Walking helps you tone your muscles, build endurance, and burn some of the maternal fat stores that developed during pregnancy in order to help you lose excess weight. These combined effects will help combat post-partum back pain, especially with the addition of basic strengthening and stretching exercises designed to restore the balance between strength and flexibility of the muscles throughout your body.

ISOMETRIC EXERCISES

Isometric exercise is a way to build muscle strength without putting stress on the joints. When performing an isometric exercise, the muscle you are targeting contracts, but your body doesn't move. For example, if you pull your abdominal muscles in tight, the abdominals are contracting, without bending the spine. Given that no joint movement occurs, the chance of injuring the unstable spine or pelvis is very low. Therefore, isometric exercises are safe and beneficial in order to restore optimal muscle strength to the spinal and pelvic muscles. The major muscle groups to focus on are the abdominals, buttocks, inner thighs, front thighs, and upper back. Hold each contraction for 5–7 seconds; repeat 5–10 repetitions, 3 times a day.

The technique to perform each isometric exercise is described below:

- **Abdominals:** pull the stomach muscles in tight, without holding your breath. If you had a Cesarean delivery, you should get clearance from your physician prior to beginning any abdominal strengthening.

- **Buttocks:** squeeze the buttocks together.

- **Inner thighs:** place a pillow between your knees and gently squeeze your knees against the pillow to tighten the inner thighs. If you have a separated pubic symphysis, this exercise may be uncomfortable since the inner thighs connect to the pubic bones. You should discuss your condition with your health care provider prior to performing this exercise.

- **Quadriceps (front thigh muscles):** sit or lay down with both legs straight. Press your knees straight down to tighten your thighs.

- **Upper Back:** Squeeze your shoulder blades together and press your chest forward.

The isometric exercises are easily done while feeding your baby or chatting on the phone with family and friends. They will help firm and tone the above muscle groups, prepare your muscles for more strenuous exercise in six weeks, and help build stability around the vulnerable spine and pelvis.

KEGEL EXERCISES

Remember these? Even if you didn't do them throughout your pregnancy, it is not too late. Beginning Kegel exercises the day after you give birth will help restore the strength of these muscles in order to provide good pelvic support and prevent incontinence. Particularly if you had a vaginal delivery, these muscles will need to be exercised daily to restore normal function and help manage post-partum pain.

Initially, it may feel difficult or uncomfortable to contract these muscles, but be persistent in your efforts and perform your Kegels daily. Start with short duration contractions, holding only 1–3 seconds, and try to perform 10 repetitions, 3 times a day. After a week, try to hold the contractions for 3–5 seconds, and perform 10 repetitions, 3 times a day. After 2 weeks, hold the Kegel for 7–10 seconds, and perform up to 10 repetitions, 2–3 times a day. Once confident with the basic Kegel, you may progress to the "elevator" variation. You will notice a gradual improvement in your ability to contract the pelvic floor, which will also help you return to your normal sex life more quickly. (Yes, eventually you will find the time again.)

GENTLE STRETCHING

All of the stretches that were recommended during your pregnancy are safe to resume gradually post-partum. If you try to stretch too quickly or too far, you may feel pain due to the instability of the pelvis and spine. Slowly and gently stretch to the point of a comfortable pulling sensation. Hold the stretch for 15-20 seconds and repeat 3 times. You may notice certain muscles feel especially tight as a result of decreased activity, labor positions used, or strain during labor. It is important to regain normal flexibility in order to minimize stress on the joints of the spine and pelvis. It is equally important to perform the stretches without experiencing pain; if you notice pain with a particular stretch, don't stretch as far, or try a different position for stretching.

POSTURE AND BODY MECHANICS

Now that you've had your baby, don't revert back to poor posture and body mechanics. It is as important now, and throughout life, to continue to work on using good posture and neutral spine alignment during everyday tasks. This will keep your spine healthy, prevent injury, and minimize any back pain you may be experiencing.

It is not uncommon for women to develop upper back and neck pain post-partum. This can often be attributed to the new positions you assume while feeding, holding, and diapering your newborn. The mother tends to look down at her little one, and this repetitve forward bending of the neck and upper back can be straining. Attempt to maintain good posture of the upper spine and perform the neck stretch, chin tuck, and thoracic spine stretch between these activities. In general, take care when performing the following activities post-partum:

- **Feeding:** Sit in a comfortable, supportive chair that allows you to rest in neutral spine posture. You may benefit from placing a pillow in the small of your back to help you sit straighter. If breastfeeding, you can use a specially designed nursing pillow to support the baby and your arms, or you can cradle the baby keeping your arms supported on the chair or pillows. If bottle-feeding, place a pillow under your elbow for support. Your shoulders should be relaxed, not shrugging up towards the ears. Although you will naturally tend to look down at your child during this bonding time, try to keep your head up to minimize neck and upper back discomfort.

- **Holding and Carrying:** Keep your baby centered along your midline to avoid unnecessary twisting and bending of the spine. Newborns can be held with both of your arms cradling them against your belly. Try not to look down excessively to minimize neck and upper back strain. If you carry your newborn in a car seat carrier, try to hold it with both hands in front of your body. As your baby gets heavier, consider leaving the car seat in the car or connecting it into the stroller to decrease stress to your spine. As your baby gets bigger and can hold his head with better control, you may choose to sling one hand between his legs with him facing away from you, again keeping him centered with your body. Front wearing baby carriers may be another comfortable option, but be careful to stand with a straight spine when using one of these. As your baby gets older, it's very common to carry her on one hip, which creates uneven forces on the spine. If you do this (and we all do), alternate on which hip you carry her.

- **Diapering:** As described for brushing your teeth, it is better to bend your knees to diaper your baby than to bend at your waist. If your neck is painful, alternate which end of the changing table you place your baby's head. You will consequently vary which way you turn to look down and balance out the positions you assume. If you use a bed or couch for your changing surface you should kneel on the floor rather than bend from a standing position.

- **Bathing:** When bathing your newborn in an infant tub, stand as close to the tub as possible and place it on a surface that allows you to stand relatively upright. When your baby transitions to the big tub, kneel at the side of the tub on one or both knees and keep your back as straight as possible.

- **Lifting:** The same rules of lifting discussed earlier apply post-partum. Always keep your back straight, hold the baby very close to your body, and lift with your legs. When lifting your baby in and out of the crib, lower the crib rail to decrease the height of the lift. Lifting your baby in and out of the car can be awkward; try your best to maintain a neutral spine.
- **Playing:** Play at eye level with your baby. When he has tummy time, lay on your belly facing him. When she plays in her baby seat or learns to sit, sit on the floor in front of her. If baby lies on his back, play on all 4's over him. Playing at eye level varies your posture, allows you to maintain better spinal alignment, and allows baby to enjoying looking at her favorite face.

You can apply the body mechanics principles I described to all of your daily activities to optimize posture, health, and comfort throughout life.

Six Weeks Post-Partum

At your 6-week post-partum check-up, your health care provider will likely give you clearance to exercise. If you have been increasing your walking, performing isometrics, and stretching, you will likely make an easier transition back to your normal workout routine. If you typically don't exercise, this is a great opportunity to start incorporating regular exercise into your life so you will be able to keep up with your child who will be running around before long. Remember that until your muscles regain full strength and flexibility, you may have difficulty performing certain activities, such as running, kickboxing, or tennis. Don't get discouraged. If you persevere, you will notice that every day you can push yourself a little harder, and eventually reach your fitness goals.

If you continue to experience back or pelvic pain at your 6-week follow-up, it is important to discuss this with your physician in order to avoid developing a chronic problem. You may benefit from professional treatment by an orthopedist, physical therapist, chiropractor, massage therapist, or other specialist. Just as back pain should not be an accepted part of pregnancy, it should not be accepted during motherhood. You have a little one who is going to keep you busy and active, and you need to be up for that challenge.

~12~

Recommended Daily Programs

A lot of information has been presented on the various exercises that can be performed to help manage and prevent back pain during pregnancy. This section provides simple, organized exercise plans that can be completed in a 40–60 minute session on any given day. Each program consists of a cardiovascular, strengthening, and stretching component. Sample plans are provided for each trimester including post-partum, and for people with different types of back pain. Given the time constraints that most people have, the sample plans do not incorporate each and every exercise. You can vary which program you follow on a daily basis for a more comprehensive and varied routine. Further, if you only have 20 minutes, you can do a condensed cardiovascular, strengthening, and stretching routine. Some exercise is always better than none.

PROGRAM #1: FIRST TRIMESTER

Cardiovascular Total time — 20–30 minutes
Walk, jog, or bike at a moderate pace

Strengthening Total time — 10–15 minutes
*Perform 2 sets of 10 repetitions for each
of the following:*

- Pelvic tilts with arms overhead holding a
  3-pound weight (p. 47)
- Pelvic tilts with leg marching (p. 48)
- Bridging (p. 52)
- Ballet squats (p. 57)
- Bent over row with a 5 to 8 pound weight
  (p. 53)
- Quadruped opposite arm and leg lifts (p. 51)
- Kegel exercises (p. 53)

Perform for 30 seconds, 1–2 times

- Deep squat (p. 58)

Stretches Total time — 8–10 minutes
Hold for 20 seconds.
Repeat 2–3 times on each side.

- Supine hamstring stretch (p. 67)
- Supine piriformis stretch (p. 65)
- Quadriceps standing stretch (p. 69)
- Sitting adductor butterfly stretch (p. 63)
- Pectoral stretch (p. 72)

PROGRAM #2: SECOND TRIMESTER

Cardiovascular   Walk, elliptical or bike for 20-30 minutes at a mild to moderate pace

Strengthening   Total time — 10–15 minutes
Perform 2 sets of 10 repetitions for each of the following:

- Pelvic tilts in quadruped or standing (p. 46)
- Wall squats (p. 55)
- Ballet squats (p. 57)
- Bent over row with 5 to 8 pound weight (p. 53)
- Quadruped opposite leg lifts (p. 50)
- Kegel exercises
  Regular and elevator variation (p. 53)

Perform for 20 seconds, 1–2 times each
- Deep squat (p. 58)

Stretches   Total time — 8–10 minutes
Hold for 20 seconds. Repeat 2–3 times on each side.

- Sitting hamstring stretch (p. 68)
- Sitting piriformis stretch (p. 66)
- Kneeling psoas stretch (p. 70)
- Standing inner thigh stretch (p. 62)
- Side waist stretch (p. 71)
- Back stretch (p.61)
- Pectoral stretch (p. 72)
- Wall posture (p. 86)

PROGRAM #3: THIRD TRIMESTER

Cardiovascular Total time — 20–30 minutes
Walk, elliptical or swim at a mild to
moderate pace

Strengthening Total time — 10–15 minutes
Perform 2 sets of 10 repetitions for each
of the following

- Pelvic tilts in quadruped or standing (p. 46)
- Ballet Squats (p. 57)
- Quadruped opposite arm lifts (p. 50)
- Quadruped opposite leg lifts (p. 50)
- Kegel Exercises
  Regular and elevator variation (p. 53)

Stretches Total time — 8–10 minutes
Hold for 20 seconds
Repeat 2–3 times on each side

- Standing hamstring stretch (p. 68)
- Sitting piriformis stretch (p. 66)
- Psoas stretch with chair (p. 70)
- Standing adductor stretch (p. 62)
- Back stretch (p. 61)
- Neck stretch (p. 74)
- Pectoral stretch (p. 72)
- Wall posture (p. 86)

PROGRAM #4: 1– 3 WEEKS POST-PARTUM

Cardiovascular Total time — 5–15 minutes
Walk at a mild pace; gradually increase time
and distance.

Strengthening Total time — 10–15 minutes
*Perform 2 sets of 10 repetitions for each
of the following*

- Pelvic tilts in supine (p. 45)
- Isometric abdominal contraction holding
  5 seconds each (p. 94)
- Isometric buttock squeezes holding
  5 seconds each (p. 94)
- Isometric inner thigh squeezes holding
  5 seconds each (p. 95)
- Isometric quadriceps squeezes holding
  5 seconds each (p. 95)
- Isometric upper back squeezes holding
  5 seconds each (p. 95)
- Kegel Exercises (p. 53)

Stretches Total time — 8–10 minutes
Hold for 20 seconds.
Repeat 2–3 times on each side.

- Standing hamstring stretch (p. 68)
- Standing adductor stretch (p. 62)
- Standing quadriceps stretch (p. 69)
- Back stretch (p. 61)
- Pectoral stretch (p. 72)

PROGRAM #5: 3–6 WEEKS POST-PARTUM

Cardiovascular Total time — 10–30 minutes
Walk at a mild to moderate pace; gradually
increase time, speed, and distance.

Strengthening Total time — 10–15 minutes
*Perform 2 sets of 10 repetitions for each
of the following*

- Pelvic tilts with arms overhead
  holding a 3 pound weight (p. 47)
- Bridging (p. 52)
- Ballet squats (p. 57)
- Wall squats (p. 55)
- Bent over row with 3–5 pound weight (p. 53)
- Kegel Exercises
  Regular and elevator variation (p. 53)

Stretches Total time — 8–10 minutes
Hold for 20 seconds.
Repeat 2–3 times on each side.

- Supine hamstring stretch (p. 67)
- Sitting "V" adductor stretch (p. 64)
- Standing quadriceps stretch (p. 69)
- Supine piriformis stretch (p. 65)
- Back stretch (p. 61)
- Pectoral stretch (p. 72)
- Wall Posture (p. 86)

PROGRAM #6: NECK AND UPPER BACK PAIN

Cardiovascular   Total time — 20–30 minutes
Walk, elliptical or swim at a mild to
moderate pace

Strengthening   Total time — 10–15 minutes
*Perform 2 sets of 10 repetitions for each
of the following*

- Pelvic tilts in quadruped (p. 46)
- Bent over row with 5 to 8 pound weights
  (p. 53)
- Quadruped opposite arm lifts (p. 50)
- Chin tucks (p. 87)
- Kegel Exercises
  Regular and elevator variation (p. 53)

Stretches   Total time — 8–10 minutes
Hold for 20 seconds.
Repeat 2–3 times on each side.

- Standing hamstring stretch (p. 68)
- Sitting piriformis stretch (p. 66)
- Psoas stretch with chair (p. 70)
- Sitting "V" adductor stretch (p. 64)
- Back stretch (p. 61)
- Neck stretch (p. 74)
- Pectoral stretch (p. 72)
- Thoracic Spine Stretch (p. 73)
- Wall Posture (p. 86)

PROGRAM #7: LOW BACK, SI, AND SCIATIC PAIN

Cardiovascular   Total time — 20–30 minutes
Walk, elliptical or swim at a mild to
moderate pace

Strengthening   Total time — 10–15 minutes
*Perform 2 sets of 10 repetitions for each
of the following*

- Pelvic tilts in quadruped and standing (p. 46)
- Ballet Squats (p. 57)
- Wall squats (p. 55)
- Quadruped opposite leg lifts (p. 50)
- Kegel Exercises
  Regular and elevator variation (p. 53)

Perform for 20 seconds, 2–3 times
- Deep squats (p. 58)

Stretches   Total time — 8–10 minutes
Hold for 20 seconds.
Repeat 2–3 times on each side.

- Standing hamstring stretch (p. 68)
- Sitting piriformis stretch (p. 66)
- Psoas stretch with chair (p. 70)
- Standing inner thigh stretch (p. 62)
- Side waist stretch (p. 71)
- Back stretch (p. 61)
- Pectoral stretch (p. 72)
- Wall Posture (p. 86)

PROGRAM #8: ACUTE PAIN

If you feel too uncomfortable to exercise, these gentle movements and stretches can help reduce pain and muscle spasm. If you experience increased pain upon attempts to exercise, discontinue and contact your health care provider.

Warm-Up   Use moist heat, soak in warm bath, or sit or walk in pool for 10 minutes

Strengthening   Total time — 3–5 minutes
Perform 2 sets of 10 repetitions for each of the following.

- Pelvic tilts in quadruped, sitting, or standing (p. 46)
- Kegel Exercises (p. 53)

Stretches   Total time — 10–15 minutes
Hold for 20 seconds. Repeat 2–3 times on each side. Choose whichever stretching position is most comfortable. For example, if sitting is not painful, perform the sitting variations of the stretches. If standing feels more comfortable, perform the standing variations.

- Hamstring stretch (p. 67, 68)
- Piriformis stretch (p. 65, 66)
- Psoas stretch (p. 69, 70)
- Adductor stretch (p. 62–64)
- Side waist stretch (p. 71)
- Back stretch (p. 61)
- Pectoral stretch (p. 72)
- Neck Stretch (p. 74)

PROGRAM #9: PUBIC SYMPHYSIS PAIN

Cardiovascular Total time — 20–30 minutes

Bike or swim at a mild to moderate pace

Strengthening Total time — 10–15 minutes

Perform 2 sets of 10 repetitions for each of the following

- Pelvic tilts in quadruped or standing (p. 46)
- Wall squats (p. 55)
- Bridging (p. 52)
- Bent over row with a 5 to 8 pound weight (p. 53)
- Quadruped opposite arm lifts (p. 50)
- Kegel Exercises
  Regular and elevator variation (p. 53)

Stretches Total time — 8–10 minutes

Hold for 20 seconds.

Repeat 2–3 times on each side.

- Sitting hamstring stretch (p. 68)
- Sitting piriformis stretch (p. 66)
- Standing psoas stretch with chair (p. 70)
- Pectoral stretch (p. 72)
- Back stretch (p. 61)
- Wall posture (p. 86)

PROGRAM #10: GENERAL PROGRAM

Cardiovascular   Total time — 20–30 minutes
Swim or pool walk at a mild to moderate pace

Strengthening   Total time — 10–15 minutes
*Perform 2 sets of 10 repetitions for each
of the following*

- Pelvic tilts in quadruped or standing (p. 46)
- Traditional squats (p. 56)
- Ballet Squats (p. 57)
- Quadruped opposite arm lifts (p. 50)
- Quadruped opposite leg lifts (p. 50)
- Chin tucks (p. 87)

Perform for 20 seconds, 2 times each

- Deep squat with 10 Kegel squeezes (while in squat position for 20 seconds) (p. 53, 58)

Stretches   Total time — 8–10 minutes
Hold for 20 seconds.
Repeat 2–3 times on each side.

- Standing hamstring stretch (p. 68)
- Sitting piriformis stretch (p. 66)
- Kneeling psoas stretch (p. 70)
- Sitting adductor "V"stretch (p. 64)
- Side waist stretch (p. 71)
- Back stretch (p.61)
- Neck stretch (p. 74)
- Wall Posture (p. 86)

PROGRAM #11: THE 10 MINUTE PROGRAM FOR LOW BACK, SI, AND SCIATIC PAIN

Cardiovascular Total time — 5 minutes
Brisk walk

Strengthening Total time — 2–3 minutes
Perform 2 sets of 10 repetitions for each of the following

- Pelvic Tilt Supine or Quadruped (p. 45, 46)
- Kegel exercises (p. 53)

Stretches Total time — 2–3 minutes
Hold for 20 seconds.
Repeat 2–3 times on each side.

- Standing hamstring stretch (p. 68)
- Back stretch (p. 61)
- Wall Posture (p. 86)

~13~

Author's Notes

I hope this book is a useful tool for you during your pregnancy. Due to the multitude of changes happening within the pregnant body, back pain tends to be a common complaint, and the techniques described throughout this book are a simple way to bring you comfort and relief during such an exciting and stressful time. The recommendations for cardiovascular, strength, and flexibility training paired with good posture and body mechanics is a recipe for back pain management not only during pregnancy, but also during any phase of life where back pain may be a problem.

Post-partum, exercise will help get you back to your pre-pregnancy weight and into shape more quickly so you can keep up with your active child. Exercise will also help energize you, and is an excellent way of relieving stress on days when your little one is testing you or pushing you to your limit. Being pregnant with my second child and chasing a very active 16 month old, I feel relieved that I got back into shape and have the stamina that I do. I am able to bond with my son while taking power walks to the playground, stretching on the floor while building block towers, and doing my squats as I make his lunch. Creatively working exercise into the day makes it easier to be consistent with my exercise routine, and allows me to cook, clean, write, read, or even relax while he naps.

I hope you utilize the information in this book to empower yourself during your pregnancy. A pregnancy without back pain is what you should strive for, and can be achieved with some work and determination. If you are not successful, your health care provider may have additional recommendations for management or may refer you to a specialist for an individualized treatment program. Everyone is unique and consequently responds differently to various forms of treatment. I encourage you to find a program that will be most effective for you personally.

I wish you much success in your endeavors for a healthy, pain-free pregnancy, and happiness and fulfillment throughout motherhood.

NDEX